Surviving Alzheimer's

Practical tips and soul-saving wisdom
for caregivers

PAULA SPENCER SCOTT

EVA·BIRCH MEDIA

For Dad, Gram, Louie, Emily, and Don,
and all those we miss due to dementia

PRAISE FOR SURVIVING ALZHEIMER'S

"Regular doses of Paula Spencer Scott's supportive and instructive wisdom should be prescribed to every family member dealing with Alzheimer's. Her Why-This, Try-This approach is a winner. It's like a first-aid kit for stressed families."

—Lisa P. Gwyther, MSW, LCSW, associate professor, Duke University School of Medicine and director, Duke Family Support Program; co-author of The Alzheimer's Action Plan

"Every bit as good, if not better, than The *36 Hour Day*, long considered the Bible on dementia care. This book is better organized and contains more detailed steps for area that often cause caregivers real problems, such as bathing. It is well researched and written in a clear, easy-to-ready style. This is my new hand-out for my clients."

—Ann Eichenberger, owner and operator of the dementia-care business Daily Dementia Caregivers in Washington DC

"Paula Spencer Scott has a gift; she is one of the rare people who is able to write about complex medical topics and make them interesting and clear. In this book, she takes on one of the quiet crises of our time, the increasing number of people who are doing all they can to care for someone with dementia. All dementia caregivers need help. This book is a wonderful gift to the millions of families on the dementia-care treadmill."

—Kenneth Robbins, MD, MPH, clinical professor of psychiatry, University of Wisconsin, and geriatric psychiatrist

"Knowledge is power in the fight against memory loss and Alzheimer's Disease. In *Surviving Alzheimer's*, Paula Spencer Scott combines her years of experience with information-packed, easy-to-read—and most important, truly meaningful—words of wisdom from herself as well as countless experts. This is a must-read for anyone impacted by the stress of caring for someone with Alzheimer's."

—Richard Isaacson, MD, director of the Alzheimer's Prevention Clinic, Weill Cornell Memory Disorders Program at New York– Presbyterian / Weill Cornell Medical Center

"Extremely thorough. I've read so many books on Alzheimer's and dementia related diseases and 90 percent of them were memoirs, not even coming close to covering the information that I needed. This book truly covers almost everything you need to know for dementia care."

—*Gary Joseph LeBlanc, founder of the Alzheimer's/Dementia Hospital Wristband Project and former* Tampa Tribune *columnist*

"*Surviving Alzheimer's* is full of good advice and helpful hints. I am so glad that there is real help now for families who are on the journey of dementia with loved ones."

—*Virginia Bell, MSW, creator of* The Best Friends Approach to Alzheimer's Care *and "The Alzheimer's Disease Bill of Rights"*

"As a longtime geriatric social worker specializing in dementia and now as a family caregiver, I looked at this book from two perspectives. It's beautifully written, covers a great deal of ground, and has many practical ideas for coping with the many changes that occur during the dementia journey as well as with the emotional upheavals of caregiving. I highly recommend it."

—*Beth Spencer, lecturer, University of Michigan School of Social Work*

"A treasure trove of practical information, addressing so many of the real-world questions and problems that I see dementia caregivers struggle with every day. This is a well-researched book that synthesizes the knowledge and experiences of a diverse group of experts (not the least of which is Paula herself) into clear explanations and actionable advice. A great choice to recommend to patients and families."

—*Leslie Kernisan, MD, MPH, geriatrician and caregiver educator, BetterHealthWhileAging.net*

DOZENS OF 5-STAR AMAZON REVIEWS:

"The book I will recommend from now on to friends beginning this arduous journey. I have a small library of books on Alzheimer's. However, this book literally had it all in a very clever format. The "what to do" section at the end of each topic is filled with great ideas. On each page, I recognized some aspect of life with my mom."

"Chock full of useful and helpful information and support. Made a difference in my life as a caretaker immediately and continuously. Provided me with a much better prospective on what and why ALZ sufferers feel and act. Everyone dealing with caregiving, at every level, can benefit from reading this book."

"The book description is totally accurate: Practical and soul-saving. I found it to be one of the most helpful books for caregivers that I have read. A must read for a stressed-out life."

"The tone is sensitive and compassionate but not cutesy or overly sentimental. The author has clearly been there and knows what she's talking about and doesn't soft-pedal the difficulties caretakers face. A must-read for dementia caregivers."

"Very, very helpful. I can't say it enough. Author teaches compassionate care, tricks, creative ways to solve problems and more."

"I could not put down Paula Spencer Scott's *Surviving Alzheimer's* and had no desire to skip any chapters. Her book provides you with excellent advice, helpful hints, options for dealing with concerns."

"I love this book! It is indeed very practical. When I'm dealing with a new situation on this Alzheimer's journey, I can easily find the chapter on a specific situation, then read why a particular behavior happens and ways to handle it."

"This book has saved me from so much stress. You learn the code to speak with them."

CONTENTS

WHY I WROTE THIS BOOK
In a nutshell: Helpers need help, too.

When the first shoe dropped, I wasn't yet thinking about Alzheimer's—at least, not in a personal sense.

At the time, I was building the Alzheimer's channel for what was then a pioneering new website, Caring.com. My specialties as a journalist have always been health, family, and women's concerns. I'd co-authored five books with doctors, been a columnist for two national magazines, and written countless articles on these subjects. So the site's mission—to provide family caregivers with support and eldercare information—appealed to my longtime interests in both academic and professional ways.

That was back when I still had two relatively healthy parents.

Or so I thought.

It's about my parents.

"I just thought you should know," my mom called to say, in the same casual tone she usually said things like *How are the kids?* and *I got a good deal on yarn today*, "that I fell and broke my pelvis and pubic bone." Since I was cooking dinner and helping a child with homework while juggling the phone, I wasn't quite sure I'd heard right.

"You don't really need to come up," she added. That was momspeak for, *Help!* My parents were in their early 80s. Of course I went up, from where I lived in North Carolina back to my childhood home in suburban Detroit. My brother Paul also came up from North Carolina to help. (The other three siblings, in three different states, would take later shifts, not that we yet realized a need for it.)

It took a day for us to set up a temporary downstairs bedroom in which Mom could recuperate.

It took half a day for the other shoe to drop—discovering the extent to which she'd been covering for Dad.

Sure, his memory had been a little spacey lately. He'd always had a bit of the goofy, absent-minded professor in him. Though he'd been moving more slowly, he still golfed and bowled. He was the longest continuous member of his General Motors bowling league, since 1948. He still sent us all snapshots of his tomatoes and hibiscus flowers that he'd printed himself from his computer, didn't he? Big travelers, our parents liked to make road trips from one child's home to the next. The videos Dad had begun taking of the passing highway, mile after uneventful mile, while Mom drove, might have been a warning sign. But he was just getting older, right?

So we told ourselves.

It's one thing to see someone with cognitive trouble for a few days as a guest in your home or at quick, chaotic family celebrations. Actually living with him in his home is a whole other plane of reality check. When my brother and I arrived, the dryer was clanking so angrily that Paul went straight to the basement to investigate. "Oh, it's just gotten loud," said Mom. (Paul found black oil pooled beneath it.) While using their landline, the connection kept shorting out. (Paul later discovered a wiring problem.) Minutes later, I punched 2:00 into the microwave to heat water for tea. The machine worked, but the number display didn't. All these were unthinkable lapses for Dad, a mechanical engineer who was such a home-repair geek that I didn't realize until my 20s that professional plumbers and electricians even existed.

And that was just the first half hour. Heating up dinner, I noticed signs of a huge grease fire under a stove burner. ("Oh, your dad was making soup and got distracted.") The next morning, Dad seemed surprised to see me: "When did you get here? Are you in town on business?"

That was a Sunday. We took him to church. "How nice to see you! Where's Eleanore?" asked my mom's best friend.

"Oh, she hurt her side and she can't walk too good," Dad told her.

"Um, she broke her pelvis and she can hardly walk at all," I clarified.

I began to learn how many meaningful conversations you can have just by meeting gazes and raising eyebrows.

Dad forgot his standing Monday golf game. His old buddy Bob pulled me aside when he came to pick him up, while waiting for him to get ready. "He's getting worse, isn't he?" he said, tapping his forehead meaningfully.

The real kicker came on day three, when from her makeshift bed Mom announced that Paul and I were to take Dad to his urology checkup. "It's just a follow-up. But you need to write down everything the doctor says because your father doesn't always pay attention lately." She didn't mention that he also might not know the current year as he filled out his intake form or that he wouldn't be able to tell the difference between a credit card and his insurance card at reception.

The urologist was surprised to see a co-ed crowd in the exam room. By this point, my brother and I had decided all three of us should be there. Dad seemed to have no objections, even to changing into an exam gown in front of me.

"So," the doctor began, "have you decided whether to go ahead on the surgery?"

All three of us stared blankly.

"The biopsy. For the mass."

What mass?! What biopsy?! Dad was oblivious, and it seemed that Mom hadn't understood the seriousness of these terms during their last visit.

The mystery mass would turn out to be kidney cancer that would kill my father in a few years—although the unsuccessful surgery later that summer to retrieve a biopsy proved so hard on Dad that we never found out for sure. Mom wisely refused to let the doctors put him through the stress of trying again, and Dad, when asked how he felt about it, merely shrugged. As happens with many people, his dementia fog grew denser after this surgery.

Meanwhile, Mom, the one with the broken bones that had launched this odyssey, wasn't doing so well herself. As she mended, I saw her lose patience with Dad's endless repetition, his habit of saying "hello, hello, HELLO?" into the TV remote instead of the phone. Having also lost significant hearing, she'd shout at him in exasperation. More discreet, astonished glances between Paul and me.

The few weeks of nursing her made it clear that my parents' days of living independently were numbered. One of us had to stay with them until Mom was back on her feet. Dad simply couldn't help her, and we were terrified of him driving. I'd heard enough frightening stories of people with dementia forgetting to buckle up, getting lost, or confusing the gas pedal and the brake. (Once a GM test driver, he must have sensed his ability was declining because he was docile about our jumping in the driver's seat, as my Mom had been doing.)

But then what? How long could things stay in this new "normal" after she recovered or in a patched-up semblance of "normal"? What if something else were to happen?

The churning conversations began. I'm not sure any of us (myself included, despite knowing the most about Alzheimer's) fully grasped how wide the ripples of the downward spiral of dementia would be, how taxing it is on any caregiver, let alone an 80-year-old partially deaf wife in dubious shape herself. One sibling thought maybe we were overreacting. Another lobbied for wait-and-see. We entertained various eventual scenarios: Move in with me? A nice place near you? Assisted living?

"Oh, we can't move!" Mom said, quashing all of it. "It would kill your father!"

Flash forward less than a year. I'll never forget the sight of my smiling, widowed dad sitting poolside in shorts and black socks on a hot North Carolina spring day, my brother's dachshund in his lap and a beer in his hand as he watched 10 of his 14 grandchildren splash about. Six months after the phone call announcing she'd broken her pelvis, my mom died of a recurrence of an earlier ureteral cancer, supposedly "cured." It had spread before it could be detected or treated. She got sick after Thanksgiving and was gone by Christmas.

That left my family, like so many families—like my Mom had initially had tried to do on her own—to figure out how to manage Dad's rapidly failing memory, odd behaviors, and childlike dependence. How to keep him busy but safe? How to keep him calm and happy? How to cope with our own conflicting levels of denial, frustration, impatience, and grief?

It's about other relatives.

We'd been through a version of this a few years earlier with my beloved maternal grandmother. Gram had been like a third parent to the five of us kids, living just a few miles away throughout my childhood, a fixture at every family party or school event, large or small. She died of Alzheimer's at 99, a very long goodbye that had ended in a nursing home.

My mom was her only child. I'm convinced the stress of caring for her mother without much help or much understanding of the disease hastened Mom's own death just three years later.

This isn't a fluke thing: Elderly caregivers have a much higher mortality rate than non-caregivers, research shows. They experience much higher depression rates, and their self-care is worse, a perfect storm for another unhappy ending. My mom was already run ragged by the time she'd begun covering for my dad, taking over more and more of the finances, driving, social planning, and other tasks. First she was a caregiver with the added burdens of being older and an only child, then fate threw in the special stressor of watching her spouse's cognitive decline, an experience that's emotionally cruel in a way an adult child can't begin to imagine.

Meanwhile, at about this same time, my mother-in-law was having similar symptoms. She would die of Alzheimer's within months of my father. (My poor four kids lost all three living grandparents, all they'd ever known, in one swoop.) In this family, too, siblings who were spread out across the country (and internationally) reacted in different ways, each according to his unique relationship with her. One wanted to dive in and solve all problems immediately and aggressively. Another moved more covertly, providing support in more subtle ways. There was massive disagreement about how she should be protected and what should happen to her home. Some still don't speak.

The stress of dementia care isn't just day-to-day. It snakes across state lines and family trees. Stigma is huge. In my mother-in-law's family, there was reluctance to suggest this matriarch might have any hint of senility, no matter how outrageous the symptoms, and especially to discuss it publicly.

Later I divorced and remarried, and, coincidentally my new in-laws also developed forms of dementia. Enter more worried and geographically widespread siblings, more medical issues, more care challenges, more divided chores and divided opinions.

After this mother-in-law died in Maine, her husband of 65 years moved cross-country into our home in California. My father-in-law taught me the true meaning of an idea I'd often heard experts express: that if you've seen one case of dementia, you've seen one case of dementia.

Unlike my other relatives, his memory remained largely intact. Instead we dealt with many new symptoms and issues caused by what we came to learn was frontotemporal dementia—delusions, talking to himself, hallucinations, being a victim of financial phone scams, and a personality-changing loss of inhibitions that meant we might find him sitting in the garden in his underwear or hear him making crude comments to my daughter's teenage friends.

He could veer from a charming, seemingly normal conversation full of incredibly remembered details to utterly wacky or inappropriate confusions quick enough to give us aural whiplash.

Those new issues—and the whole new level of caregiving stress the experience ushered in—inform this revised edition. I've also added more about topics readers have expressed interest in hearing more about: ways to communicate better, an explanation of the "Why-This, Try-This" approach, more on specific symptoms and resources, and an extensive new chapter on end-of-life care (intended to be read at any point in the disease because, as wrenching as it is to think about, foreknowledge helps).

It's about you.

Ultimately, I wrote this book because millions of family members touched by dementia are living through similar stories.

While working at Caring.com, I personally experienced everything the website covered then: not only coping with Alzheimer's and cancer care but also navigating sensitive family relationships; arranging financial and legal paperwork; working with gerontologists, social workers, attorneys, and physicians; researching housing options; cleaning out a longtime home; relocating an elder; working with hospice; finding out how to write an obituary and a eulogy. My personal arc reached from "uh oh" shoes dropping to unstopped grief.

And as I researched topics like these for the site, these experiences became layered with new wisdom. Each time I covered an academic meeting on aging or gerontology, gave a talk, or conducted an interview, I learned more. For six years, I worked with remarkable MDs, PhDs, MSWs, and an alphabet soup of other experts, as well as countless un-credentialed but often equally knowing hands-on caregivers.

Surviving Alzheimer's summarizes these insights and practical solutions in a way that's speedy and accessible. That's because few of us have a lot of time and energy, even as we have tons of questions, worry, and stress.

Alzheimer's and other dementias don't just strike a person's brain; they strike his or her whole support network. If you're like me and my family, you'll often feel at sea. *Surviving Alzheimer's* is the resource I'd have wanted to help me get safely to the other shore.

o o o

NOTES ABOUT THIS BOOK

If someone in your life has Alzheimer's or another form of dementia, you probably want to know things like:

- What should I say the twentieth time I hear, "What time is it?"

- Is there a way to make bathing less stressful?

- Why does he or she wear the same clothes day after day (or rummage in drawers, make things up, or fly off the handle, or—you name the odd behavior) and what, exactly, can I do about it?

- How can I keep this person occupied today in a way that won't stress me out?

- How can I get this person to accept my help?

- How can I get my family members to help me?

- Is it normal to be so stressed? Constantly?

- And, wait, what's the difference between Alzheimer's and dementia, anyway?

You want answers and insights quickly, as questions come up. Although more information exists on Alzheimer's and other forms of dementia than families could find just a generation ago (thankfully!), accessing what you need when you need it can be a pain. It takes effort to sift through long pages of explanation or to scan scores of web pages and forum threads to figure out what's reliable and then pull out the "gems" that will actually make a difference in your everyday life.

Adding to the challenge of sorting out optimal dementia care is that there are so many different perspectives. Each expert has a particular vantage point, informed by his or her unique training and field (or personal) experiences. Neurologists, for example, explain what's going on in the brain and what might alter it. Geriatricians offer medical guidance. Mental-health experts shed light on personality and relationship changes. Social workers, occupational therapists, gerontologists, nurses, safety experts, nursing-home workers, palliative-medicine specialists, and researchers of all stripes have studied or developed the best approaches for different aspects of care and everyday life. Not least by far, experienced laypeople have their own hard-won personal caregiving stories that can instruct and inspire.

Surviving Alzheimer's sifts through the best of these diverse insights and "connects the dots" between their perspectives. From those many dots, I've drawn a road map to help you navigate terrain that constantly winds through surprising new vistas and stressful hairpin curves.

Theory is fascinating. Narratives are important. But nothing cuts stress like applying fast, clear, realistic, and practical collective wisdom that works.

A Few Words About Semantics:

"Alzheimer's" I've deliberately chosen to refer to Alzheimer's in this book's title because that's the word that most people know, and it's the number-one cause of dementia symptoms. Alzheimer's is named for the German doctor, Alois Alzheimer, who first identified this disorder in 1906. (Don't we all wish his name had been shorter and easier to spell?)

Much is unknown about the causes and process of Alzheimer's—researchers don't even agree that it's a single disease. We now do know that brain changes can start two or more decades before your friends first notice you're repeating comments and have trouble balancing your checkbook (pre-clinical or pre-symptomatic Alzheimer's).

Mild cognitive impairment (MCI) refers to a stage of disease where changes in thinking skills are growing obvious but don't yet interfere with daily life. But not all cases advance to Alzheimer's. As problems progress, many cases called "Alzheimer's" are thought to be triggered in part by vascular problems (such as small strokes), or dementia symptoms are caused, or worsened, by other health problems such as depression, diabetes, or alcoholism.

Other forms of dementia emerge as different parts of the brain degenerate. And because there's still no reliable, easy, and widely available way to get a certain diagnosis for what we currently call Alzheimer's, many people never really know for sure what's causing their dementia symptoms.

We just know Mom forgets to turn off the stove. Bob crashed his car again. Granddad has begun talking to things that aren't there. Jane needs help choosing clothes, paying her bills, cooking, bathing, managing her pillbox. And we step in.

Although there are obviously some nuances specific to, say, Parkinson's dementia or dementia with Lewy bodies, the advice in this book can apply to different kinds of progressive dementias.

"Loved one" Two more prickly words: loved one. Sometimes I use this phrase to describe the person with dementia. I'm well aware, though, that it's not always the case that the person being looked after is a beloved figure. Sometimes they're estranged spouses, parents, stepparents, or in-laws with whom we have fractious or indifferent histories.

Unfortunately, we don't have a crisp word for "person with dementia" or "the person in your care," since *caree* and the chilly *care-recipient* aren't widespread—at least, not here in the U.S. So sometimes I go by the majority who do love their relative with the disease and call that person *your loved one*.

"Caregiver" Finally there's this word choice open to interpretation: *caregiver*. Most of us don't describe ourselves this way or think of ourselves this way. Even with a confused 95-year-old living in our home, for whom we did all the meal prep, financial management, medical advocacy, and nearly all of his daily and end-of-life care, my husband and I didn't think of ourselves as "caregivers."

The word is how researchers and academics refer to family members who look after someone with dementia, but research shows that laypeople tend to think the word refers to those who are paid to do the job.

We tend to just think of ourselves as daughters and wives, sons and husbands, friends and family, simply doing what needs doing.

I get that. But I use the word caregiver anyway because it's apt and shortish and because, frankly, we don't have a better word. (*Carer* never took off outside the U.K.)

Helping someone with Alzheimer's is one of the more stressful undertakings a human being can be thrust into. You can climb mountains in less time. You have more training for driving a car. You get more support when you download computer software. Unlike other tough jobs, there are no paid vacations or glowing reviews. Unlike the similar selfless routines of raising a baby, there's no diploma, wedding, or other happy marker of a job well done to look forward to.

I know this. And I'd like to make it a little easier for the MILLIONS of us struggling to stay afloat.

Please Send Your Feedback.

Are there subjects missing that you wish had been included? Do you have a tip or tactic that has worked for you that you'd like to share, in the hopes it can help another family?

Please help others who are dealing with this disease by sending your ideas or comments to survivingalz@gmail.com

Thank you.

** All of the names in the caregiver anecdotes in this book, other than my own (noted with the initials P.S.S.), have been changed, and some stories are composites.

o o o

"Devote what energies you can muster to being kinder, more understanding, more loving to those who are still on this earth and to whom you are responsible. And save some for yourself, because you will need it."

—Jerald Winakur, MD, in *Memory Lessons: A Doctor's Story*

1: THE BIG PICTURE

Insights and inspiration from the Wizards of Alz

We all crave fast answers. That's why the bulk of this book contains practical, problem-specific, what-to-try-now tips and ideas.

But first things first: When dealing with the sometimes maddening behaviors and situations that Alzheimer's brings, having an overview that guides you through the forest—and not just around each confounding tree—can dramatically cut your current and future stress.

That's why I've included this section of bigger-picture principles from the people I've come to think of as the Wizards of Alz, each of them amazing in his or her own way.

Here, meet some of the best thinkers in dementia care. Each carefully chosen expert shares a perspective that's been shaped by his or her in-the-trenches experiences. Together, these views weave a strong foundation for your thinking and your actions as you navigate this new world you've entered.

o o o

Bob DeMarco: Step Into Alzheimer's World

While caring for his mother for 8 years, a son discovers a life-changing epiphany: Changing your attitude changes everything.

When Dorothy DeMarco died of Alzheimer's disease at age 96, hundreds of condolences poured in from around the world to her youngest son, Bob. "Dotty" wasn't an international bigwig. She was the muse, star, and object lesson of a blog that Bob had started to help himself understand his mother's condition after he moved to Delray Beach, Florida, to become her full-time caregiver. ("The world's biggest support group," he calls it.)

That blog, Alzheimer's Reading Room, is now a leading voice and information source for Alzheimer's caregivers, with thousands of followers. Bob, a former business executive and Wall Streeter who took care of Dotty for 3,112 days, continues sharing the lessons he and others have learned as the site's editor. And if you think his posts are rich with inspiring, eye-opening tales, you should get him started talking, as I was lucky to do.

Most of the things caregivers experience at the start are negative reinforcement—you hear things like "Nobody survives" or you see how stigmatizing Alzheimer's can be. Everything seems to be going wrong, and you can't even control your own emotions.

I spent my first 18 months as a caregiver trying to get a handle on what was happening. I'd stay up 'til 3 a.m. reading about the brain. I tried to adjust my life to take care of my mom. All my friends had always loved Dotty, but she had turned meaner than a junkyard Doberman Pinscher. She'd resist me, argue with me, curse me.

Classic example: Dotty would open the freezer and stand there. She'd look through the food, open up packages, maybe re-wrap some. Meanwhile the freezer would start this incredibly annoying beeping, an alert to let you know you'd left the door open.

"Ma, what are you doing?" I'd yell from the next room.

"None of your damn business!" she'd holler back. We'd go back and forth awhile. Then I'd go in to close the door myself. She'd throw down the package she had in her hand and go curl up in a ball in her room. Things like this were happening every day.

Something has to change! That's what I found myself doodling on a notepad late one night. I circled the words and stared at them. I had no idea what it meant. But I felt the stress start to come out of my neck. I didn't even know I'd been that stressed. A few minutes later, I wrote:

And that something is me! I circled those words, too, and then I connected the two phrases with a line. I still wasn't sure what it all meant, but I went to bed feeling unusually relaxed.

I'd made all our interactions about me—me being annoyed by the beeping, me getting mad when she wouldn't take a shower, me trying to tell her she just ate when she said, "I'm hungry." I thought I understood her confusion and was changing my life to deal with the effects of Alzheimer's. But it was all still about me. My mother was only going to change as the disease did. It dawned on me: What had to change was me—my reactions, my actions, my words, my emotions.

I had to enter Dotty's world—"Alzheimer's World," as I've come to call it.

If I'd had a travel guide to Alzheimer's World, these are some of the tips I wish had been in it:

- **Use the local transportation**. Before I interacted with my mother, I'd take a step to the left—literally take a step, as if I were walking into a new place. I did this to re-train my own brain to remember I had to enter my mother's world.

- **Speak the local language**. Eventually I realized I was drowning my mother with too many words. Sometimes, all I needed to do was smile. Or put my arm around her shoulder and my head on her head. Instead of a long explanation about what we were going to do (like go to the bathroom before lunch), I'd stick out my hand and say, "Let's go."

- **And she'd come along willingly, even before asking**, "Where are we going?" To which I'd just smile and say, "To have fun." Little did she know that I was the one who was going to have the most fun, after she took a pee without a fight about it!

- **Stick to a routine**. Structure the day to replace bad patterns with good patterns. Build on what the person did before. My mom used to get up, read the paper over coffee, and run around on errands. So we'd do the same thing, only we'd go to McDonald's or sit outside, because I found that the bright light seemed to help her mood. We'd go to the gym, where the exercise made her smile and that brighter look on her face would last for an hour or two after.

- **Never forget you're in a new place**. So many people get hung up on thinking, "You're not the person I used to know." But that objectifies the person and distances you. It's saying, *you're a problem* instead of *we're in this new place together*.

So here's what I did about that annoying freezer beep: I stayed calm and took a step to the left. I tried to figure out why my mother might be rummaging around in there. I realized that her whole life, she'd open the freezer to look for something to cook later. But then she'd forget what she was doing. It was comforting to see it this way. Or maybe she was hungry but couldn't discriminate between the fridge and the freezer. She'd open the freezer, but nothing there was edible. Also, she either couldn't hear the beeping or, if she could, she didn't know what it meant, so it didn't bother her.

So I put a box of donuts, a treat she loved, in the back of the freezer. The next time she went in there, she found it, took out two donuts that were frozen together, closed the freezer, and set the donuts on the counter. Later, she came back into the kitchen, saw them there, and ate them happily—without opening the freezer.

Instead of venting—calling my friends and telling them the same story over and over—or getting bent out of shape and angry, I became proactive. Instead of feeling burdened, I felt a kind of joy that Dotty was still using her brain to find something to eat.

Each episode like this brought the positive reinforcement I needed as a caregiver that my efforts were worthwhile—and I wanted to do more of it. The better I became at living with Dotty in Alzheimer's World, the more pleasant and cooperative she became. She still had her pain-in-the-butt days, but they began to bother me less. Something else surprising happened: I became more patient and easygoing in the Real World, too. Small stuff bothers me less. Let's face it, positive reinforcement motivates all of us.

o o o

Lisa P. Gwyther: Blame the Disease, Not the Person

Fear? Denial? Disagreement? This co-founder of the Alzheimer's Association knows better than most that families must navigate an ever-changing "new normal."

What led Lisa Gwyther to create some of the first-ever dementia support groups, newsletters, and other educational resources for families about Alzheimer's? "They simply didn't exist when I started, and they were needed," says the director of the Duke Family Support program and education director of Duke's Bryan Alzheimer's Disease Research Center. A social worker with four decades of experience in aging and Alzheimer's services, Gwyther is also an associate professor in the Duke University Medical Center Department of Psychiatry and Behavioral Sciences. She was one of 30 co-founders of the national Alzheimer's Association and is a past president of the Gerontological Society of America.

"Knowledge is power," is one of her many truisms—and the earlier you identify and understand memory loss and other symptoms, she believes, the better. I've often heard Gwyther, an inspiration to many in aging services, quoted at conferences. She and I "met cute": Out walking one morning, I recognized her—from her author photo on her excellent book, The Alzheimer's Action Plan, *written with Duke's P. Murali Doraiswamy, MD, and Tina Adler— coming toward me. I'd interviewed her many times by phone without realizing she was my neighbor!*

The disease affects everyone differently. If you've seen one family facing Alzheimer's—well, you've seen one family facing Alzheimer's. And the disease and families change over time, bringing new behaviors, symptoms, conflicts. Other unexpected things happen, meaning each "new normal" is only normal for so long.

People are surprised to hear that there's no one "right" answer or way to do things. There are too many variables involved. There are usually as many "right" ways to make a decision as there are families. You can only do what seems best at the time, in a situation often limited by circumstances beyond your control.

What trips up families most: They get mad at the person with Alzheimer's for the frustrating things he or she does or says and the personality changes they see. Or families get mad at each other for disagreeing about what to do, for not helping enough, for being too cheap or being too critical—you name it. But it's the disease they should be getting mad at. The disease is what's making their family member act in frustrating, intrusive ways and demanding so much of everyone involved.

Put up a reminder sign for yourself that says, BTD! ("Blame the disease!") It doesn't help to try to get the person with Alzheimer's to act differently or to extract promises about future behavior; he can't. You, not your relative, need to change.

There are no perfect families. All families disagree or have regrets sometimes. Most families disagree often. Alzheimer's can draw a family together or tear them apart.

Support groups offer something for almost everyone. Early stage support groups can be a relief and inspiration to people recently diagnosed (and their care partners). They're often social and supportive, as well as educational. Other groups are just for spouses, or for daughters only, or men only. People are sometimes skeptical or suspicious about groups at first, and it can be hard to get away to attend. But support groups provide a kind of compassion and camaraderie where everyone there "gets it," sometimes in ways family and friends just don't. Some groups meet online.

Support groups aren't for everyone. I've seen older men, for example, who respond better to the idea of attending an information session or seminar, like those hosted by hospitals or the local Alzheimer's Association. They're valuable, too. Some people aren't the type; they fear support groups will be like group therapy and force them to talk (which isn't true).

How to identify a good support group: Sit in on one, and listen for lots of "Ah!" and "You, too?"

Families talk about saving for a rainy day. Well, if you're dealing with Alzheimer's, it's pouring. Be sure you're seeking the appropriate level of care. Early in the disease, that can mean extra structured activities or in-home supports. Later, a common mistake is to think assisted living is the only answer, when the person with dementia may benefit from an adult day program or may need a secure dementia-care facility or skilled nursing care.

3 mantras to help you stay sane:

1. The disease is bigger than me. Define your limits, then call in reinforcements.

2. Let's focus on what's left, not what's lost. People with Alzheimer's have a lot to give.

3. I did what seemed best at the time. Don't waste limited energy second-guessing yourself.

o o o

Teepa Snow: Decoding the Secret Language of Dementia

The woman who might well be called the "Rosetta Stone of dementia-speak" offers insights on what it means when a loved one says, "I have to get home," and more.

No one falls asleep at a lecture given by Teepa Snow, an occupational therapist and dementia-care consultant with more than 35 years of experience. She slips into character and invites the audience to role-play at her popular training and education workshops for professionals and family caregivers. Her goal: to drive home the lessons she's learned working with stroke, brain injury, and Alzheimer's patients, including her own grandparents. ("Although back then," she says, "they just said Grandpa was senile.")

Developer of the Positive Approach to Care, Snow works with organizations across North America and teaches at Duke University's School of Nursing and the University of North Carolina–Chapel Hill School of Medicine. While she was waiting for a plane one August afternoon that would take her to her 245th presentation of the year (she logs 300 travel days a year), I caught up with her on the subject of what the baffling words and actions of someone with dementia can mean.

Behavior "talks" to you. Instead of getting mad or frustrated because the person with dementia acts inconsistently or nonsensically, try seeing the behavior as a message. A behavior is like the tip of the iceberg—something to be curious about, to investigate and to explore, rather than to judge.

Say your frail dad starts to rise from his chair. "Don't!" you yell from across the room, "You'll fall!" He's telling you *this seat is not agreeing with me*. Or, *I need something*. Or, *I see something*. When you yell for him to stop, you're not helping. Without meaning to, you're making him feel bad (or sad or mad or scared), and he doesn't understand why. So he tries again. And again, you say, "Don't!" He tries again, and you come over to gently push him back. He grits his teeth and says, "No, no, no, no, no!"—and finally, he hits you! Out of nowhere!

But it didn't come out of nowhere—he gave you lots of warning. Better to think, as your dad starts to get up, *Hmmm, what can he see from there that caught his eye? Is he thirsty? How* *long has he been there? Is his arthritis bothering him?* Think through what unmet needs he may have.

Communicating is like a treasure hunt. Too often, we want to get to the prize without having to go through the scavenger hunt of collecting clues to get there.

That's really hard for family members, especially, because we rely on old patterns to guide behaviors and communications. We also tend to have an agenda—we just want to fix the problem. We don't follow the other person's agenda, which is affected by the dementia. We rush to do things that need doing without understanding how it seems from his or her point of view.

We have to slow *way* down to communicate.

We're most comfortable getting messages across with words (and to a lesser extent, intonation). But with dementia, you lose vocabulary and comprehension. You hear fine, but by the middle stage of the disease you only understand every fourth word. Imagine that I nod my head at you and say what sounds like (let's take away the consonants) "Aeouoi ie?" You might automatically nod your head back and say, "Okay," in a kind of social chit-chat way. And then you just sit there. But I was saying, "Are you coming with me?" And you didn't move! Your words and actions didn't match! As caregivers, we assume the message is getting through. We can't quite grasp that someone with dementia is no longer following those usual rules.

Always start with a positive physical approach: Connect first, then go to your "agenda." (Greet, then treat!) Don't charge in and say, "Mom! Your shirt is on backwards! What are you doing? Let's fix it. It's time to leave for lunch!" Better: Make friendly eye contact. If you open your hand near your face and then offer it to the person, it cues her to look there, at your eyes. She'll notice your hand and realize you want to come near and be with her in a friendly, familiar way.

When you get close, turn your body sideways, while keeping your face toward the person. (It's called a supportive stance, as opposed to a confrontation stance.) This way, she can see you're paying attention, but you're not "boxing her in." Get to her eye level. Sit or kneel (if she's sitting) or stand if she's standing. Say something like, "Hey Mom, it's Teepa." One thing at a time.

Then take a second to make a quick assessment: Is this a good moment or a bad one? Does she recognize me right now or seem aware of who I am? If not, she won't be very excited for me to start tugging her shirt off. It's about being respectful.

If she does seem aware, you can point to your shirt first, then hers, letting her eyes follow your gestures: "Oops, Mom, looks like you might have a coffee stain." Now gesture a "come on" signal, then say, "Let's go get a fresh one, and put this in the wash."

Try to avoid the words "LET ME HELP YOU." It makes it sound like you think the person is incompetent.

If she seems distressed, sad, or upset, address that: Match your facial expression to hers and then say, "It looks like..." "It sounds like..." "You seem...." Be empathetic to make the connection before moving onto your agenda.

Five magic words: "Tell me more about that." People with dementia often have trouble coming up with the right word. They tend to get stuck at the noun. Imagine you wanted to use the word *coconut*. But you can't come up with it. You might describe it: "Like Almond Joy, like Mounds, the stuff in there." People with dementia not only can't find the right word, they tend to lose nouns first. So they might say: "Round hairy ball brown stuff." I think, *Hmmm, something yucky?* I'm not going to hit on coconut.

Now imagine if I said, "Tell me more about that."

"Hairy in the brown ball!"

Oh, *in* the brown ball. I might say, "Show me that." Or, "Show me what that does." Or, "Show me how you use that."

You open your mouth. Ah! And I can ask more questions, like, "Do you eat it?"

Same thing with phrases you don't understand. A common one is *that baby*. "That baby needs help." It means, "I need help" or "I have an unmet physical need" or "I have an unmet emotional need." Another phrase used a lot, *I've got to get home* or *I want to go home*, means "Something's not right—I'm hungry, thirsty, lonely."

Repeat the comment and ask about it: "You've got to get home? Tell me more about that. Is there something you need to do there?"

"No, Mama's there."

"Tell me about that. Is there something you need from her?"

"I need to ask her what to do." Ah! This tells you she's not sure what to do or she's bored.

Tell me about it is a great decoder phrase: Tell me about that baby. Tell me about home.

Say she repeats, "I've got to go home, I've got to go home," over and over in an agitated way. You can tell from the tone and delivery that it indicates acute distress. She's not processing you or anything around her. In this instance, you could repeat what she's saying, following her rhythm: "You've got to go home? You've got to go home?" You telegraph that you get what she's saying, you get that she's upset. You connect.

Another break in the usual system of communication: People with dementia often get too close or touch too much. They might come over and rub their hand on your shirt. You say, "Mom, why are you touching me?"

"Because you're pretty and I like you," she answers. She likes it, so she touches it or she takes it. She doesn't understand that it isn't hers. She lacks that filter.

Or she sees a child she likes, so she starts talking to him and patting his body. You say, "Mom, stop that!"

"But I'm just trying to be nice," she says. "He's cute."

"Mom, you can't touch him!" It's hard not to judge that kind of behavior, but try not to sit in judgment. Understand that she's trying to navigate the world around her and having a hard time doing so. When you point out her mistakes, she gets flustered.

Caregivers tend to fall into the habit of seeing what's wrong. They point out what's wrong, trying to be helpful when the person with dementia is making mistakes: Uh oh! No, no, don't you remember? Remember I told you? Remember you agreed? The word "remember" has no place in your conversation. They don't remember. They can't, so why point it out and cause friction?

Dementia isn't just a memory issue. If you just think "memory," you're denying the devastation the person is trying to live with. The person is suffering from brain failure, in two ways:

1) Structural failure, which means parts are broken and can't be fixed, and 2) Mechanical failure, where the wiring fritzes out—now it works, now it doesn't. That's why five minutes ago, it was, *I know who you are and why I need a walker*. But now it's "Who the hell

are you and get out of my face with that walker!"

People with milder stages of dementia often have the hardest time because they still have awareness and memory present. They think, *I hate feeling stupid! I'm not a stupid person!* For some, the greatest distress is the thought that *nobody knows what I'm going through*.

They're doing the best they can with what they have left. Our challenge is to do the best we can to try to match up. Your flexibility is critical. Let go of how she was five minutes ago. You'll have more success—you'll be less stressed—if you can be in the moment and try not to judge. ("What a temper! She's fooling with me on purpose—she knows she needs her walker!") They're not doing things on purpose or to make you mad!

Trying to see it the way they're seeing it turns everything around.

o o o

Ken Robbins, MD: Be an Advocate, Not an Adversary

A geriatric psychiatrist explains how you can avoid those all-too-common damaging conflicts, arguments, and battles of wills.

With his training in psychiatry, internal medicine, and public health, and a clinical practice specializing in geriatrics, Kenneth Robbins, MD, has been my go-to source for countless eldercare topics: stress, depression, burnout, resistance, anger, sexuality, incontinence, aging fears, grief, and more. My favorite collaboration (and one of the most popular with readers) was a series of articles on how to talk to aging parents about difficult or sensitive topics. Whatever the subject, Dr. Robbins has the gift of being able to absolutely "get" (and explain) the needs of all the affected parties as he moves people from "stuck" to solution.

A clinical professor of psychiatry at the University of Wisconsin-Madison, and board-certified in psychiatry and internal medicine, Dr. Robbins speaks and writes frequently on psychiatry and the law, dementia, depression, anxiety, and suicide risk and prevention.

If you're dealing with dementia, you're probably going to run into arguments and conflict. You should just expect that, at times, your patience will be severely taxed.

There's a long list of reasons why: People with dementia often require constant attention, and that makes it difficult to get basic tasks accomplished—including sleep! What's more, the person with dementia is likely to be difficult to get along with at times. He's likely to have limited insight into his illness and therefore may resist necessary safety measures, for example. Most people with dementia also struggle with psychiatric difficulties, in addition to their cognitive limitations. Depression, anxiety, or psychoses are likely to make them very uncomfortable and irritable at times.

On top of all that, other family members or friends are likely to have their own ideas of how the person with dementia should be cared for, even though they're not the hands-on caregiver. Hands-on caregivers often struggle with social isolation. The combination of the incredibly hard work, a lack of appreciation from the person with dementia and often even from family and friends—plus sleep deprivation—will leave even the best caregivers overwhelmed at times. It all makes it difficult to avoid conflicts.

If your relationship was already contentious, caregiving makes things all the more complex. When you start out resentful, it's harder to have empathy, easier to quibble. But even if you had a good relationship, there's more conflict as your loved one becomes more self-absorbed and says things he or she normally wouldn't. It happens to almost everyone.

A common, sad scenario: As someone changes, he says things he normally wouldn't, nasty things: "You never cared about me! You always think of yourself first!" And the caregiver is stunned. She says to herself, *I thought we had a good relationship. Maybe that wasn't real—he was just being polite all these years!*

Almost always, though, what's said in the moment does NOT reflect how the person with dementia has always thought. As the disease progresses, the person becomes more self-absorbed. As he loses more and more brain cells, he loses the capacity for empathy, much like a young child. If his needs aren't met in the moment, he lashes out with what he's feeling in that moment. It's not a broad commentary on you or your relationship. Too often, this wrong interpretation is what the caregiver remembers after the person dies.

All people with dementia become self-absorbed. You can't take what they say or do personally, because they no longer have the capacity to focus on anything beyond their own needs, much like a young child.

You never win an argument with someone who has dementia. The reflexive way we all talk, when you believe your point of view is more correct, is to try to reason. But you can't compete by the old rules because you're not on the old playing field. The other person is completely self-absorbed and no longer capable of abstract thinking. No matter how reasoned your side is, it's extraordinarily rare that by explaining the reasons why something is unsafe or unwise, you'll convince your loved one.

Better: Talk about feelings. "You want to drive your car? Wow I can tell how much you miss being able to get around whenever you want. It must be hard. Let's talk about some ways you could get to the diner and the places you want to go." Acknowledge the feelings but avoid being an adversary. Gently redirect to safe choices.

The challenge is how to negotiate without becoming the enemy. If you're going to help, you need to be perceived as being helpful. Anytime you feel strongly that a behavior is unsanitary, unsafe, or otherwise problematic, it's wise to get a third party involved. This sidesteps nagging and arguments and instead gives you the ability to take the role of supporter, helping the person follow someone else's advice. That's easier with some big things, like driving or needing to move to assisted living, where the logical person to take the hit is the doctor. That frees you to empathize: "I sure wish you could stay in your home but the doctor says it's just not safe. I'm so sorry, but we have to follow what the doctor advises." Make clear that you're on your family member's side.

It's more of an ongoing struggle during the day with smaller things that are dangerous or not appropriate—the husband for whom chewing has become difficult but still wants steak, or the mother who wants to light candles, or the person who keeps feeding the dog over and over.

The obstacle caregivers face is that conflict can be continuous. It's your job to protect the person with dementia, so you have to say there are certain things he can't do. Try to arrange your life so you're not always the "no" person. Give "yes" choices you're comfortable with: "We don't have any steak today, but I can give you your favorite pasta."

A lot of people never get this new way of communicating because it's so unnatural! We spend our lives with someone having logical discussions together, reasoning things out. It's hard to stop! Your parent or spouse looks the same, but his or her brain isn't the same. You have to develop communication skills that are probably completely outside of your experience.

Endless conflict can slide into depression for a caregiver. Caregivers are twice as often depressed as non-caregivers.

Everyone needs to feel appreciated for all they do, but the person with dementia isn't capable of giving that kind of feedback. It's no longer a truly reciprocal relationship. Caregivers run ragged if they don't have other people to talk to for emotional support.

Here's something that happens more than you'd think: The caregiver brings the person with dementia to the doctor's office and tells him or her all the things that are going wrong. Under the circumstances, it seems natural for the caregiver to sound tired, irritable, and pessimistic. The doctor thinks *heck, I'd feel the same way in that position*. But the doctor doesn't realize that the caregiver is in fact depressed, and that's why she's so negative and having such a hard time.

One of the cardinal symptoms of depression is anxiety and problems with sleep. You wind up impatient and just not able to be there for the person you're taking care of.

When you're depressed, you're not capable of being a functional caregiver. Learn the warning signs of depression and be persistent about telling your own doctor (as well as your loved one's) about your symptoms. Being a caregiver is one of the most challenging things a person can do. If you're depressed, that makes it nearly impossible.

o o o

Amy Goyer: This, Too, Takes a Village

Having the right support can extend your ability to keep going, AARP's expert on multigenerational issues knows—not least, from caring for her own live-in parents.

Amy Goyer knows what it's like when your dad can still physically dress himself but can neither locate nor identify the underwear that you must hand to him. She knows what it's like to put off dental checkups for two years because you just don't have time, even though your teeth hurt (and wind up needing two new crowns). After years of long-distance caregiving—flying between her home in Washington, D.C., and Phoenix, where her parents lived—Goyer relocated to Arizona in 2009 to be nearer them. In 2012, she began looking after them in their home. She's gone through everything from pneumonia scares and insurance battles to feeding-tube care and not always being recognized by her dad. (He now has advanced-stage Alzheimer's; her mom, who had heart disease, died at age 87, in 2013.)

And that's just Goyer's personal life. As AARP's longtime Family and Caregiving Expert, she's a spokesperson, popular speaker, and blogger who also consults with other nonprofits and corporations. In typical working caregiver fashion, she wrote her second book, Juggling Life, Work, and Caregiving, *by staying up until 4 and 5 a.m. for far too many nights. As she once told NPR's Jackie Lyden during a radio appearance, "I'm not just trying to keep my parents alive. I'm trying to have a good life with them and live my life at the same time."*

You don't see yourself as a caregiver when you're starting out. I'm just a daughter, helping Dad. I'm a spouse helping my husband, or my wife. That's one of the biggest deterrents to getting support. "Caregiver support" sounds too official to apply to you. But if you're calling your parents long-distance to check on them or help with their finances, you're a caregiver. If you're doing what I'm doing as a live-in provider of care every day, you're a caregiver.

There's a huge range of us. And we all need help!

Isolation creeps up on you because you don't have time or you're too tired to do the things you used to.

Our normal support systems don't always adapt to our being a caregiver. I have friends who help me out with projects or with yard work. But intensive caregiving? You can't truly understand, deep in your soul, what it's like until you've been there. The people around you don't know. They aren't vigilant about urging you to get out or take a break. They don't know how to help. They get tired of listening to you vent or say, "I can't believe that just happened!" Caregiving truly separates out the dedicated friends and family members.

The biggest deterrent to getting any help is that we're moving too fast! We're constantly bombarded with needs and issues and crises. There doesn't seem to be any time to stop and find support. Yet that's exactly why we need to see the value of it.

My doctor just warned me that I'm in adrenal fatigue from burning myself out—and I should know better! Like many caregivers, I thought my parents were so much more vulnerable than I was, so they needed all the help. Also there's a tendency to think nobody can care for your loved ones like you. This is true. It's also true that you can't do it every second. You have to take the risk to let someone else take part.

We tend to view help and support as selfish. It's not just "doing something nice for yourself." We need energy to provide care—just as our cars can't run on empty, neither can we. It's practical, not selfish, to re-fill our own tank. Anything that helps us ultimately makes life better for the person receiving our care. Dementia care is often a long, slow decline—and without lots of help, we wind up in a slow decline, too.

One of the most underutilized kinds of support is direct help for caregivers. When certain mundane tasks are done for me, like yard work, errands, cleaning closets, sorting mail, that frees me up to do more of the things I want to do for my parents. When I was looking for someone to check on my house when I'm out of town, I discovered what's called a personal concierge, or personal assistant. What a lifesaver!

The first reaction is always, "I can't afford that!" But for $15 an hour, one hour a week, I know something that I'm stressing about will get done. For $15! And that lowers my tension and stress. (Rates vary by market.)

Some other great sources of support that people aren't always tuned into:

- **Your local Area Agency on Aging**. It's the #1 place to call. (See "Resources.") They should be able to refer you to most of the agencies and resources in your community.

- **Home-based medical care**. Getting a loved one somewhere can be a huge ordeal. People don't realize that doctors who make house calls still exist. There are also mobile x-rays, mobile EKGs, ECGs, ultrasounds—all done at your home.

- **The Veterans Administration (VA)**. My dad is a World War II vet, but he wasn't tied in to the system. It's true that it took a year and arduous paperwork. But now he receives VA "Aid and Attendance" cash pension benefits, which are designed for veterans and surviving spouses who need regular assistance for care. He also receives help with bathing and housekeeping, as well as respite care, through the VA. The VA also has a caregiver helpline (855-260-3274).

- **Respite care**. A colleague once cautioned me against using this term because people might not know what it means. I think it's more likely that most of us don't know how this feels! Respite care is when someone else temporarily looks after your loved one so you get a break. Adult day services are an overlooked resource for this; some specialize in dementia-care. You may also be able to find short-term stays in assisted living or nursing-care facilities. And some states have voucher programs where you can choose someone to provide respite for you, such as a neighbor or friend, and a grant covers that short-term care. Or, as I found out, your relative may qualify for respite through Veterans Affairs.

- **Supportive therapies**. I'd be remiss not to mention music therapy, because I started out as a music therapist. I've never come across someone I couldn't connect with through music—and having your loved one occupied allows you to get a break. There are other specialists, too. For example, I hired the swim instructor from my parents' former senior community to work with my dad (and me!) in our pool. It was great exercise and cognitive stimulation for him—and me!

If you're working, be up front with your employer that you're a caregiver. Many people are afraid to share this. We're taught not to mix business with personal matters, not to bring home into the workplace. We fear we might not be seen as committed or reliable. But for the most part, it's better for your employer to understand why you're coming in late or taking time off—and you'll be better able to tap into resources and benefits your company might offer.

Start by talking to human resources. Ask what benefits and policies might affect you as a caregiver, including flexibility on hours, leave possibilities, and employee assistance programs, such as discounted legal assistance if you need to seek guardianship or a power of attorney. Ask how to talk to your supervisor about it.

Be very clear that, "I'm committed to my job," and then, without giving too much information, tell them the gist of your responsibilities. Don't overlook things at the workplace designed to support your health, like exercise facilities, gym discounts, or counseling services.

There's one more kind of support caregivers who've been there often credit for their survival, though it's not often talked about: spiritual support. So many caregivers describe this as a spiritual journey, in the sense of a life-lesson journey. They say that faith is the thing that gets them through always being on the edge of the abyss, feeling you'll never get it all done.

Spirituality helps caregivers feel good about what they're doing. It can give you the faith that, even when things don't make sense, you can keep putting one foot in front of the other.

o o o

David Troxel: Give 'Em a Reason to Get Up in the Morning

Meaningful activities improve mood, cooperation, and even cognition—but planning things to do needn't be a burden on you, says this expert on Alzheimer's therapy.

"Alzheimer's? What's that?" friends would ask David Troxel back in the mid-1980s, when he began working at the University of Kentucky Alzheimer's Disease Research Center (one of the first such centers funded by the National Institutes of Health). "There were no medications, few services, and little awareness," says the dementia-care consultant. But there was, also in Lexington, one of the first day programs for people with Alzheimer's, founded by Virginia Bell. Frustrated families would bring in loved ones, warning, "Mom's so ornery!" or "Dad won't do anything!" Hours later, having done some art and exercise, maybe set a table or talked with others, they'd leave almost as if a different person. Troxel began to focus extensively on activity-as-therapy.

In 1996, he and Bell developed the "Best Friends model" for Alzheimer's care, which holds that what each person with dementia needs most is a steady friend who will provide loving care, accept their illness, and learn the "knack" of boosting quality of life. The duo also wrote the oft-quoted "Dementia Bill of Rights." Troxel, whose mother, Dorothy, died of Alzheimer's in 2009, is a past president of the California Central Coast Alzheimer's Association.

With Bell, he co-authored A Dignified Life: The Best Friends Approach to Alzheimer's Care, a Guide for Family Caregivers *and* The Best Friends Book of Alzheimer's Activities. *Though written mainly for long-term care professionals, you'll find the two activity guide volumes dizzyingly full of great ideas, including advice on tailoring them for different stages of dementia.*

Why you don't want to flick on the TV and park your loved one: It might seem easy, but ultimately, it's not helping you or your family member. People with early stage Alzheimer's have told us they value creative activities as a tool for maintaining quality of life. All through the disease, interacting with others and doing absorbing things can improve mood, provide a sense of meaning and accomplishment—and enrich lives (theirs and yours).

Socialization is treatment for Alzheimer's disease.

Boredom is the enemy. If nothing is going on, it often leads to the challenging behaviors that we see—agitation, aggression, crying, wandering.

Current medications for memory are modest in their impact. The good news, though, is that we've learned a lot about how to help people with Alzheimer's through activities and engagement.

I'm not talking about just being generally kind and loving. It's about building pleasure into the day. Use activities as a tactical strategy to foster cooperation and success as a care partner. This kind of approach can turn a "no" into a "yes."

Dignity is key. Keep things on an adult level. I'm not for crayons or baby dolls, which can feel demeaning and lead to frustration or anger (although everyone is different and some people are comforted by dolls). Think about your parent's or partner's life story and build rituals around that. Are there parts of their life story that evoke a smile or pleasant memory? My mother, a Canadian, loved a cup of Earl Grey tea with milk, and it would soothe her on a bad day. Maybe your mom loves to talk about her childhood on a wheat farm in Walla Walla, or your dad likes to revisit his famed hole-in-one and do a little putting with you.

People often ask me, "Do you think I should...?" And I usually say, try it! Want to take Dad to a ballgame? Sure. Have a plan B—bring a pal with you to help, be prepared to leave early. But don't fear failure. There's a bit of emphasis in the world of Alzheimer's care on "failure free" activities and sticking with what works, but I think people with dementia are like the rest of us—they like novelty.

Always doing the same, safe activity can get stale and boring. It's good to be bold. (Using common sense, of course—maybe a 43-day road trip in a Winnebago isn't such a good idea!) You'll know soon enough if something isn't working. And you can regroup.

Start with categories of activities like these:

- **An ongoing project**. My all-time favorite came from a woman in New England whose mother loved ice cream. (Don't they all?!) One summer, she decided they'd visit every ice cream store in the area and create a scrapbook about it. They had their picture taken together in front of each shop, saved souvenirs like menus and napkins, and rated and reviewed each place. It was like their own Zagat guide. By the end of summer, they'd been to 23 ice cream shops and had a wonderful scrapbook to reminisce over.

- **Anything musical**. Lyrics can stay in the brain even after language skills are lost. Music can be a real source of joy. My mother loved to listen to the 40s and 50s music channels on cable TV. I'd also rent old musicals on Netflix—if you turn on closed captioning, the song lyrics pop up. We'd have a sing-along. Later, when she lived in a care facility, I'd talk up taking her to a "concert." We'd make ourselves nice to go hear, say, Luciano Pavarotti (even if it was just a CD playing in the music room).

- **Just being outside**. Take a walk, sit on the front porch, wheel your mom out in her wheelchair. You don't have to DO anything. Twenty minutes outside gives a day's worth of vitamin D.

- **Doing things for others**. When Santa Barbara neurologist Robert Harbaugh gives a diagnosis of Alzheimer's, he also tells patients, "Now I want you to go to church / go to Macy's and spend your husband's money / volunteer somewhere." He knows that being social is key. Your mom might not want to do an art project, but she'd make something for her grandchildren. One woman and her mom baked dog biscuits for local animal shelters. Intergenerational activities work on multiple levels.

- **Simple chores**. People with dementia still need to feel productive—arranging flowers, sorting and organizing, folding clothes, hammering nails. When my mother was in assisted living, I'd keep rolls of wrapping paper, bows, and supplies in her room. I kept buying new things for her to help me wrap—for a friend, I'd tell her. She had so much fun, picking the paper, holding the ribbon while I tied the bow.

- **Solicit advice**. I'd bring my mom half a dozen dress shirts and neckties, and ask for her help. She loved matching the shirts with the best neckties. It's empowering to feel you have a say in things.

- **Yes, exercise**. You already know the evidence shows it's so powerful. It may even be able to slow the progression of Alzheimer's disease. But one of the unsung benefits is that it provides small successes, a sense of accomplishment to take that short walk, or stretch with a therapy band, or do simple yoga. Bonus: Exercise builds strength and balance, reducing the risk of falls. And it's good for you, the caregiver, when you do it together.

Socialization and engagement shouldn't fall completely on your shoulders. Don't wait to tap into services near you. Look for an adult day center that has a dementia program. They're hard to find, but you're in luck if there's one near you. Or see if you can get someone with an upbeat personality to come into the house to talk and do simple projects with your relative, someone who's lively and laughs.

You don't have to structure every moment of the day. The idea is to improve your lives, not make it harder on you by being a one-person activity committee. Try to build in three or four anchor activities throughout the day, things that become part of your routine, such as a morning stretch followed by a favorite music show or nature video, time before lunch to play with or groom a pet, then afternoon tea or happy hour. When you think about your life or mine, we don't have every minute planned out. Sometimes we're busy, sometimes we nap or just sit on the sofa.

Doing nothing is also doing something. People with dementia tend to want to be with you. "Activity" can sometimes mean just being next to you while you do your own thing—going driving, going to the grocery store (if Mom isn't an aggressive wanderer), or just holding hands with you while you sit and read.

Don't overlook simple pleasures. My mom loved nothing more than going for a drive and listening to old music. Then we'd pull into a drive-through restaurant and order a hot dog followed by ice cream, so we didn't have to get out of the car and deal with waiting at a table and all that. Plus, it had all the winning elements many people with dementia seem to love—driving, music, and ice cream!

o o o

Anne Basting: Forget What's Lost, Enrich What's Left

Music, art, and telling stories can transform "sick" Alzheimer's patients into artists, says a MacArthur-winning educator.

Early in her career, having won a yearlong fellowship to study acting and aging, Anne Basting, PhD, found herself in a Milwaukee nursing home. For seven weeks she struggled to spark residents' memories in creative ways—unsuccessful until she said the fateful words, "Forget about remembering. Let's make it up." The stories they spun together became a series of plays Basting staged—and the kernel of an idea she's since taken to care facilities nationwide.

The popular organization she founded, TimeSlips, trains family caregivers and professionals in improvisational storytelling for people with memory loss. You can train yourself online at timeslips.org.

In 2016, Basting was awarded a MacArthur Fellowship—the so-called "genius grant"—for her creative, inspiring efforts to build programs that use the arts to transform the lives and communities of home-bound elders, nursing home populations, and people with dementia, among others. She has loads of great ideas and initiatives going. Her focus: changing the environment of care to focus on creative engagement, or what she calls "the cultural cure."

We have a tendency to see dementia in black and white, as if you are or you aren't. But after a person is diagnosed, he or she might well live 15 or more years. Clearly, that time is not all a meaningless void. People can have symptom-free days, hours, minutes, or seconds. Dementia is not about half full or half empty. It's not about black or white.

The experience of memory loss is gray. We need to get comfortable in the gray and keep our eyes and hearts open for moments of grace.

Memory is social. This doesn't mean visiting people more. It means reknitting them into the fabric of our lives. Too often I hear people say, "It's just too hard to be around him." "It's so hard to see her this way. I just can't go." And that is how—so simply, so gradually, so quietly—people with dementia lose their most valuable remaining thing, their circle of friends. Friendship changes with dementia for sure. But it can continue to yield gifts to both people.

The arts have an amazing power to reach people with dementia. When rational language begins to erode, symbolic emotional communication remains. That's what art is: symbolic emotional communication—sharing a vision of the world through gestures, words, sounds, images. Shared communication of any kind—through singing, dancing, visual art, poetry, or storytelling—can bring people suffering from loneliness and isolation into community.

Opportunities for creative expression allow the person with dementia to be not a patient who is sick but an artist who can grow.

Our first healing impulse is to work on memory. In the 1990s, when I was volunteering at a nursing home, I tried many memory-based techniques to get residents to engage in conversation. I got nowhere. Out of desperation, I switched to imagination—replacing the pressure to remember things with the freedom to imagine. What I learned: Lean less on memory and more on shared visions.

TimeSlips is a creative-storytelling method that grew out of that experience. It's something any family can do at home. You look at an image together and ask open-ended questions that encourage the person with dementia to imagine stories about it. Use all your senses to listen: What are her facial expressions? The gestures she uses? The sounds she makes? It also helps to echo—to play those expressions back to the person with dementia to be sure you're getting them right. (If she frowns, you frown. If she laughs, you laugh, too.) This simple act of intense, whole-body listening and confirming is an act of deep respect.

When a loved one has difficulty remembering a name, a face, a date, a story—try shifting to a shared journey into the imagination. "I wonder what the people in this picture were thinking about: What do you think?" Or, "I don't remember her dog's name, either, but if we'd had a pet, what would it be?" Just relieving the pressure to remember can open communication and connection.

You might think, "Oh, my dignified father would never go for something like that...." But you'd be surprised. People with dementia start to forget their social role. They might not remember they're a spouse, or a parent. They need a social role through which they can express who they are, and the role of storyteller really supplies that.

o o o

Naomi Feil: Focus on Feelings

You can reach through confusion to make an emotional connection, even when dementia is advanced. This insight from a pioneering therapist is a gift that's changing eldercare.

Naomi Feil, founder and director-in-chief of The Validation Institute, literally grew up among the severely disoriented oldest-old, in a home for the aged in Cleveland, Ohio, where both her parents were managers. Now in her 80s, Feil is a legend in dementia care. Her compassionate Validation Method (also known as the Feil Method) for interacting with older adults with Alzheimer's-type dementia has been widely used by professional and family caregivers worldwide since the 1960s. She's the author of The Validation Breakthrough: Simple Techniques for Communicating With People With Alzheimer's and Other Dementias.

"People hear this is a disease that gets worse and worse and there's nothing you can do," she told me. "But hey, these are human beings with human needs." To see her in action (and bring tears to your eyes), search online for "Naomi Feil and Gladys Wilson," for a clip from the PBS documentary, "There Is a Bridge."

When people are very old and deteriorated, no one enters their world. They're often just sitting there. They withdraw inward more and more, their desperate need for connection all inside. Here's a person who has worked his or her whole life, contributing their whole life, who needs that connection again to feel a sense of worth. They're longing for closeness.

Validation is a way of communicating with very old people who have an Alzheimer's-type dementia. It restores a feeling of dignity and self-worth. It's a way of being with them, feeling what they feel. You pick up their emotions and reflect them back. People who are validated feel safe.

"What's the point?" some people think. Families are told so often by the medical community that Alzheimer's is a disease that just gets worse and worse, that there's nothing you can do. It doesn't have to be that way! Even though people diagnosed with Alzheimer's lose memories and their emotions may seem gone, these are human beings, with human needs. They're not worthless.

Even with someone who appears to be in a vegetative state, you can break through.

My philosophy is that there is a humanity that binds us together. When people get very old and have advanced dementia, they go back to this basic humanity. And you can reach the person on an emotional level, because you're both human beings who share human experiences.

Family members often grow angry with their relative for behaving in ways they can't understand. Behaviors almost always have some underlying reason. The person has an unmet need. It might be to be useful and productive; to express feelings; to be listened to and respected; to resolve unfinished issues; or to restore a sense of equilibrium when eyesight, hearing, memory, or mobility fails.

People often use repetitive movements to express their needs, especially when they can't talk. Body movements replace speech. Women often sew. Men often use their fist as a hammer. Folding and refolding, such as a napkin, is also very common, and tends to represent a need to get safe and feel nurtured. Objects can mean different things for different people. For one man, I learned that touching a shoe symbolized sex with his wife. For another, a shoemaker, a shoe was about working.

Ask specific questions about what the person is doing or saying: "Will it fit?" "Is it a miter joint or a butt joint?" That shows interest and encourages a response. Use an ambiguous pronoun (like it, they) to keep it going. Specific questions with vague pronouns also are useful with someone who communicates with words you can't understand. For example, the person might say, "I wirld with the woomets." You may not understand what *woomets* are, but you can say, "Was it fun? Did they say anything?" When you ask in an interested, nonthreatening way, you get a response.

You may not learn the meaning of the action or what need is being expressed. That's okay. Sometimes you learn a lot. The main thing is that you're in communication in their world. That's a lot! The person is less isolated.

The best way to approach: First, take a moment to focus on your breathing—slow, deep—to release as much frustration and anger as possible before you interact. Use a clear, low, loving tone of voice. Harsh tones can make the person angry, and soft, high tones are difficult for many older adults to hear. Get very close and make eye contact. Eye contact shows affection and reduces anxiety.

Use words that get at facts, rather than emotions. Factual words are more nonthreatening and build trust. Ask: Who? What? Where? When? Maloriented people aren't interested in understanding why they behave the way they do. In fact, they retreat when confronted with their feelings. So rather than arguing, engage: "Who is stealing your jewelry, Mother?" "What does she take?" Draw out a conversation.

Another helpful approach is to rephrase the gist of what the person said with the same key words and same level of intensity: "You're upset about x. You want me to do y."

Events, emotions, colors, sounds, smells, tastes, and images create emotions, which trigger similar emotions experienced in the past. Old people react in present time in the same ways they did in the past.

To help ease anxiety or complaints, ask about the most extreme example of what's causing a concern: "What's the worst that could happen?" "Is that the worst x you ever saw?" Inviting deeper talk allows the person to express feelings more fully—and release them.

Match the person's motions and emotions: how they breathe, how they move their hands or legs to further enter the person's emotional world and build emotional trust. One woman, a former legal secretary, made busy finger movements in the air. Instead of ignoring the behavior, her caregiver began air-typing, too. They made eye contact. "You can type how many words a minute?" asked the caregiver. "Ninety-two" the woman said, with pride. They were the first words she'd spoken since moving to the nursing home six months earlier. The validating caregiver established empathy.

When someone feels wanted, needed, understood, there's a completeness. I know it gives me energy to connect with an old person this way, and it makes the other person feel the same.

Sometimes in someone with very little speech or no speech, you see a repetitive motion—moving the hands or rocking back and forth with the eyes closed. Maybe a tear is coming down. They, too, have a need that needs to be expressed. They've withdrawn from the world in order to nurture themselves. Approach from the front. Approaching from the side or behind can startle. Gently use touch if the person doesn't resist. Try different ways of touching; think about where a mother touches a child. For example, move your fingertips in a light, circular motion along the upper cheek. Every cell remembers where your mother once touched it.

I often use music when speech is gone. Not any song. You have to know the songs the person knew. Try singing a song from childhood. For many people, religious music, even a simple old hymn like "Jesus Loves Me" or "Amazing Grace" can be powerful, because of the emotion and safety that's tied to it. Get close and use gentle touch, and sing, matching your voice to the rhythm and intensity of their motions. If they're flapping their hands energetically, be energetic. If they're breathing soft and slow, be soft and slow. The person may begin to respond to your rhythm and touch you. You may not get a response the first time, but you might the next, or the next. Or this nonverbal person might even open his or her eyes for a moment and sing with you. You'd be surprised at the emotional connection you can create.

All this is communication. And the person is no longer alone.

o o o

Leslie Kernisan, MD: 5 Things I Wish Caregivers Knew

A geriatrician urges you to shift how you think about medical care after a dementia diagnosis. It can make a world of difference for the affected person—and you.

Knowing a doctor experienced in the care of older adults is valuable. Knowing a geriatric specialist like Leslie Kernisan, MD, who also understands family caregivers' critical role as health-care partners, is priceless. She's one of only 7,500 geriatricians in the U.S.—about 10,000 fewer than needed to meet current aging needs, and 25,000 fewer than the projected need by 2030. "As a society, we're depending more and more on caregivers to help us provide the care that older people need," she says.

Board-certified in both geriatrics and internal medicine, Kernisan makes house calls and offers geriatric consulting services to families in the San Francisco Bay Area. The former associate medical director of the Over 60 Clinic in Berkeley, California, she has a background in quality improvement, healthcare leadership, and public health, and helps teach geriatrics at the University of California, San Francisco. Not least, Dr. Kernisan (my collaborator on many caregiving articles at Caring.com, where she was a senior medical editor) writes two blogs—Geriatrics for Caregivers and GeriTech—and is the force behind BetterHealthWhileAging.net, a site providing practical information, podcasts, and webinars on senior health and family caregiving. She's also developing online courses to help family caregivers better help aging relatives with their health issues.

Wish #1: I wish dementia caregivers knew that what seem like "little things" can make people much worse. Untreated pain, constipation, too much stress, medication side effects—you don't think they're that big of a deal, but for an older adult, they can be huge. Often these "little things" make a person with dementia much more confused or difficult than he'd otherwise be.

These seemingly minor problems can even wind up sending your loved one to the emergency room or hospital, which is a stressful and risky experience for someone with Alzheimer's. And that means another crisis you and the rest of your family will have to deal with.

- **Pay attention when a new problem develops, especially if it's over hours or days**. Whether it's something physical, behavioral, or with thinking skills, don't automatically assign every change to the dementia. Make sure something else isn't going on.

- **One of the biggest problems caregivers don't always act on: sudden worsening in mental abilities**. This often indicates delirium, which means there's likely something wrong, like an infection. This is extremely common during hospitalizations or after surgery but people don't always realize that it can happen outside the hospital, too! For instance, it's not uncommon for a family caregiver to mention to me at a scheduled exam, "She's been much more confused in the past week." We often then discover a urinary tract infection or medication side effect, and sometimes find really serious medical problems underlying the new confusion. In one case, we discovered a large pocket of pus next to an elderly woman's lung, which explained her cognitive downturn. Don't wait a week. Don't wait until the next appointment you have. Call the doctor or advice-line that day, and be ready to bring her in today.

Wish #2: I wish dementia caregivers knew to have doctors re-evaluate the care plan for other chronic illnesses in light of a dementia diagnosis. Most older adults have more things going on than the dementia. You don't want to stop treating chronic conditions like diabetes or high blood pressure just because someone has been diagnosed with Alzheimer's. But many of these chronic illnesses require self-care that can get hard when you have memory loss and cognitive changes. It's often possible to be "less aggressive" in a treatment plan so that the person benefits without going through quite as much hassle or risk.

- **Common examples**: People with insulin-requiring diabetes should be given a simplified insulin regimen. It can also be hard for people with dementia to properly take "as-needed" medication, such as for pain or for COPD. Instead the plan needs to be simplified, or you need to recruit more help to keep track of how the person is doing and how often they need to take the medication.

- **It's not bad to simplify a care plan!** Most doctors can do this, but you have to ask for it because specialists, especially, are focused on the problem at hand for them. Ask, "Is there anything we can simplify to make the care regimen more doable?" Often, if this happens at all, it happens too late. That's a mistake.

Wish #3: I wish dementia caregivers would get used to thinking about the real pros and cons for every aspect of care. I call these the benefits and the burdens. Many treatments and procedures are overly burdensome to people with dementia and may be less likely to help than people realize.

- **Here's a common scenario**: Someone with dementia is found to have a mass that's possibly cancer. The doctor wants to biopsy it and, if it's cancer, offer whatever treatments are possible. You'd want to ask: "How stressful will the evaluation and treatment (if necessary) be? What would happen if we just watched it? And what are the answers to these questions in light of this person's overall health?" If the person has been in and out of the hospital over the past couple of years due to congestive heart failure, for example, then a full-blown cancer work-up may not be the right thing to pursue.

- **For any major diagnostic procedure or treatment, ask, "How will this help with my loved one's care overall?** And what are the likely burdens?" This is especially true for same-day treatments that involve sedatives or anesthesia. Often these tests and procedures are quite stressful and even risky for people with dementia, but many doctors don't focus on this when they recommend the test. So you really want to be clear on how the test results might help you better manage the person's overall health.

- **Get the doctor to help you think about the big picture of the person's health**. Doctors won't always remember to do this. Specialists, especially, tend to focus on the specific problem you've brought to their attention and how to fix it. They each focus on their own branch of the tree, and that can be to your detriment, because you need help with the whole tree. You need to know which branches to pay attention to most.

Wish #4: I wish dementia caregivers knew that it's really important to have somebody knowledgeable about the person with Alzheimer's come to the medical visits. Too often, people with mild dementia come alone. Sometimes it's because they want to highlight their independence. Or it's just plain hard for the caregiver to come in.

- **The trouble is**, people with dementia often have difficulty providing doctors with enough information, or with details on a symptom or a problem. This means important health issues can be missed or not get properly addressed. Anybody, whether you have dementia or not, can have trouble remembering what the physician says. Everybody needs an advocate with them at doctor visits—especially someone with dementia.

- **What if the person doesn't want you to come?** Try to explain that you'd be helping them retain important information. But if they won't let you, or you can't be there, you have options. At minimum, you can write up your questions and concerns and send it to the doctor before the appointment. Or you can ask the doctor to call during the visit or send back a summary in writing or via email. Another approach is to sit in on part of the visit but also to step out for a bit so that the person with dementia gets some private time with the doctor.

Wish #5: I wish dementia caregivers would start the process of advance care planning with the doctor as soon as they know they're dealing with dementia. Good advance care planning should start with conversation, reflection, and learning more about what to expect health-wise down the road. And of course, because we want the person with dementia to be as involved as possible, earlier is better.

- **To learn what to expect regarding dementia, consider watching videos online together of people with advanced dementia**. They can be hard to watch, but they've been shown to change the preferences that people express in their health planning. Be sure to consider what other health problems, besides the dementia, might bring on a life-threatening crisis or cause real health declines.

- **The hard, overlooked reality**: People with dementia often have other serious illnesses that may bring the end before dementia does. For example, someone with advanced COPD who has a bad crisis and ends up on a breathing machine won't be able to tell you his preferences, even if his Alzheimer's is mild stage. So it's important to talk about how other major diagnoses are likely to evolve, while you can both discuss them. Someone who has dementia and who's on kidney dialysis eventually won't understand why he's being held down and poked, and probably won't do well.

- **Ask for help understanding the overall health picture**. Not all doctors are comfortable helping families with advance-care planning. If yours isn't, try saying something like, "Before we do this paperwork, we'd like to review the overall medical picture and what conditions are most likely to affect him." Ask, "What might happen in the next one to two years? What key medical decisions can I be expected to have to make in the next year or two?"

- **Revisit documents as the person's health evolves**. That's especially important when there's a major change in health that changes the person's abilities (like a stroke) or health trajectory (like a cancer diagnosis). Repeated hospitalizations can also signal a time to reassess the advance directive. It's common to decide to prioritize different things as the person becomes frailer or sicker. So often I have families tell me "Oh, my mother did her advance directive 10 years ago." Well that was then! Now that she's in a different health situation, she (or her surrogate decision-maker) may have different ideas on what should be done in the event of a serious health crisis or if it seems some form of life support may be needed.

- **Of course no one likes to think about health crises and how our loved ones might die**. But in the long run, this can really reduce the stress on caregivers. One study showed that when families end up making decisions at the end of a loved one's life, the negative stress effects from factors like uncertainty and the logistics of decision making can last for months or years; advanced directives specifying treatment reduced caregiver stress. Plus, it's important to try to honor a person's wishes and preferences at the end of life. Planning gives people a way to think about those wishes, share their thoughts with loved ones, and document them so that doctors have guidance on what to do.

o o o

Barbara Kate Repa: To Protect Against Later Legal Hassles and Care Headaches, Act Now

This attorney and caregiver knows all too well that few families like to discuss the "what ifs," even if dementia is the mother of all wake up calls.

For 50 years, attorney Barbara Kate Repa has kept in touch with a dozen friends she grew up with in Wisconsin. One recent year, though, a third of them, including Repa, had to skip their annual reunion due to what they called "mom watch." Their mothers, nearing the end of life, needed hands-on care even more than the daughters needed camaraderie and wine. "So many of us are in the same situation," she says. She shuttled between Milwaukee and her San Francisco home until her mother died in 2016.

Repa's career intertwines consumer legal education and eldercare. She's an author of WillMaker, the bestselling software that allows laypeople to write their own wills, healthcare directives, powers of attorney, and final arrangements. She currently writes and speaks about eldercare issues and serves as a counselor on The Friendship Line, the nation's only suicide-prevention hotline and (for non-urgent calls) warmline serving people 60 and over. A former volunteer ombudsman (resident advocate) in memory care nursing homes, she's also a past president of the Bay Area Funeral Society and the California Board of Funeral Directors and Embalmers.

Despite her long expertise in senior legal issues, her own father, Frank Repa, had no will when he died in 2003. "Our Midwestern reserve got in the way. The dirty topic of who-got-what wasn't part of polite conversation," she recalls. "In the long run, that thinking doesn't serve anyone. And in our family, the failure to face the issue of mortality head-on created a huge mess that took months to sort out. That could have been avoided if we'd just had a couple of conversations about it."

Why this stuff matters: I see some caregivers who have all their loved ones' legal and financial matters in order, with neat sets of matching file folders. More often, people's heads are in the sand. What the ostriches don't realize, until it's too late, is that someone will have to take care of all sorts of legal and practical matters when their loved ones can't: ensuring appropriate medical care, inventorying and managing property, filing tax returns, selling assets—and, after death, distributing property as the law or estate planning documents direct.

It's relatively easy to get things in order when your loved one is still mentally competent. But it can become a BIG headache if you wait. To put it in perspective, naming an agent in a power of attorney now to deal with financial issues takes a couple hours and often involves no cost. The alternative—waiting until your loved one isn't mentally competent to sign the forms and being forced to get an adult guardianship or conservatorship—can take time, cost thousands of dollars, and also sacrifice personal privacy as matters of mental competence are aired in court.

The two things most people need to think about are:

1. Protecting money and assets (with a financial power of attorney, to handle the person's money in his lifetime if he's unable, and a trust, will, or both that will take effect after death)

2. Ensuring appropriate medical care (through a HIPAA release, so you can view and discuss medical records; a medical power of attorney, to name someone to handle decisions when the person is incapacitated; and advance directives that express preferences, so you don't have 10 different family members arguing over what "Dad would have wanted").

Even through moderate-stage Alzheimer's, people can have the mental capacity to finalize these documents. (Not that you should wait this long, if you can help it.) The law generally only requires that a person understand what the document is and what it does at the time it's finalized. We all know that the thinking skills of people with dementia come and go. They have good days and bad, and they tend to do better in the morning than late in the day.

To help protect the legal validity of these documents, there a few precautions you can take. Think about who you have as witnesses. Don't just grab whoever's in the waiting room. If capacity might be questioned later, get witnesses who truly know the person with dementia, someone who can say, "Yes, I had lunch with Joe that day and he was lucid; we talked about the past and the future."

Making videos is also becoming popular. You can record the person saying something like, "I have strong feelings about my medical care, and so I'm making these decisions." Writing a letter, if the person is the letter-writing type and can still write cogently, is another way to preserve evidence you might need down the line to prove your loved one had the required mental capacity.

Even though I believe most people don't need a lawyer to help with many end-of-life documents, it's usually a good idea to get an expert involved if your loved one has been diagnosed with Alzheimer's, especially if you suspect any document might be challenged. No lawyer should finalize a document if she felt the person lacked legal capacity to make it, so a lawyer's testimony may be helpful evidence in case of a later challenge. It's best to find someone who specializes in eldercare or estate planning for an older person, because they'll understand the key issues, from Medicaid planning to practical ways to stave off family disputes.

Biggest source of confusion: How and when these documents take effect. People sometimes think that if they're named as an agent in a power of attorney document (for healthcare or for finances) they immediately become the person in charge. They think it means that they can ramrod through any decision. But that's not true. In most cases, the document takes effect when the person is no longer able to make decisions as certified by one or more medical experts. And it only lasts until the person's death. Check the document for specific wording about how and when it takes effect. Or be sure to write one that takes effect immediately if that's what's required.

Biggest source of lasting family grudges: Disputes over money and assets. Like many other things, family fights tend to follow the money. Documents having anything to do with money and other property—wills, trusts, power of attorney for finances— are the ones most challenged, so make sure you get them right.

There may be another reason to act to protect money and other assets: fraud. Unfortunately, a lot of people prey on older adults with dementia. Lonely elders are vulnerable to a friendly voice on the phone or may fall into an old-fashioned politeness and not have the gumption to say no.

Often what's needed most is to get another set of eyes on an older person's finances just to be sure he or she is not falling for trumped-up home repair or insurance schemes that could deplete funds needed later for essential housing and care costs.

A financial power of attorney should be in place to make sure bills are paid, that forgotten bills don't turn into legal problems, and so on. The person named as the agent is often a family member, but it could be a trusted friend or even a trained outsider (like a professional fiduciary).

If you're the agent named in a power of attorney for finances, it's important to be transparent about how and where the money you're managing is spent. Make sure you fastidiously document all inflows and outflows of money. It's easy to do with Quicken or other simple financial software. Or hire a bookkeeper if you're not good at it. You want to stave off any future challenges from anyone who might claim you were acting wrongfully.

You may be able to do a lot informally to deal with finances, too. The solution may be as easy as talking with the staff at the bank to get the information needed to monitor another person's accounts and expenses. There's supposed to be an iron curtain of privacy in finances. The reality is that if your situation is a known commodity, especially in a small town or where they know your mom and dad, bank staff may be willing to set up online access for you or deliver copies of statements.

One of the great "shoulds" in life: We should all prepare a will. Yet more than 70 percent of people over 55 don't, an American Bar Association study showed. With dementia, it's a good idea to get an attorney's help to protect against future legal challenges. At home, you can start by asking the person whether he or she has ideas about specific people or organizations getting particular property.

The property covered doesn't necessarily have to be valuable. It can be something with mostly sentimental value that might get overlooked by others, such as vacation mementos collected over the years. It's a good idea to sketch out these things before you get to a lawyer's office, to save time and money.

You don't need a will or trust for everything to ensure there's a chain of ownership for property after death. A car and a bank account are the biggest assets many people own—and you can often simply name the next owner to take them by specifying a "transfer on death" or "pay on death" beneficiary. In most states, you can do this with a simple form at the Department of Motor Vehicles (DMV) for a car or at a bank for checking and savings accounts. On the owner's death, the property or money passes directly to the person designated rather than having to go through the time and expense of the probate process.

When monitoring your loved one's medical care, it's often enough to get a HIPAA release form to get access to his or her medical records. The patient is usually required to have some capacity to give access but doctors will often overlook this, especially if you're working with a geriatrician (specialist in older adults), who is more likely to bend the rules and have the attitude of "we're all in this together."

A lot of medical records are now online. If you have your loved one's access info (including a password), that's a golden nugget.

Also, encourage your loved one to complete an advance directive or power of attorney for medical care, which designates a person to supervise medical care and specify the care wanted if he or she becomes unable to express those wishes. The best help in resolving questions about such documents usually comes from medical personnel rather than an attorney, who doesn't know the person's symptoms and situation or the possible effects of various treatments. Doctors are supposed to follow all advance directives, but slip-ups happen. Sometimes family members don't know they exist, or medical personnel overlook them in a file.

As added insurance, there's another kind of medical directive, which is relatively new: the POLST (physician's orders for life sustaining treatments) or MOLST (medical orders for life sustaining treatments). The exact name given depends on the state. The benefit is that the doctor must also sign it, signifying that he or she will provide only the care the patient would want for both current and future medical treatment.

Another advantage: You can still set up a POLST or MOLST if your loved one is slipping; they don't usually require capacity. Another person can complete them on behalf of the patient.

Don't pay for documents directing medical care. The patient representative at your local hospital should be able to supply them, free. You can also find the forms online by searching your state name, "statutes," and the document you need: power of attorney for medical care, advance directive, or POLST.

o o o

Richard S. Isaacson, MD: Balancing Hope and Realism

Medicine and diet can't cure your loved one, but it's important to know how they might help (both of you!), says this cutting-edge neurologist.

Richard Isaacson eats likes he talks. That is, he follows his own advice about the increasingly promising benefits of diet and nutrition in slowing the onset and progression of Alzheimer's. At a working dinner one evening, he chooses the salmon and lots of veggies. He sticks to a single glass of red wine. He passes on dessert, although he's partial to dark chocolate, and tells me he tries to get a similar dose of beneficial antioxidants with less sugar by stirring packets of dark cocoa powder into his morning coffee.

It's not just academic for Dr. Isaacson, a neurologist with a family history of Alzheimer's who founded and directs the first Alzheimer's prevention program at a major university, the Alzheimer's Prevention Clinic, Weill Cornell Memory Disorders Program at New York-Presbyterian / Weill Cornell Medical Center. He's also an associate professor of neurology at Cornell, where he specializes in Alzheimer's disease risk reduction. His books include The Alzheimer's Prevention and Treatment Diet *(with Christopher Ochner) and* Alzheimer's Treatment, Alzheimer's Prevention: A Patient & Family Guide. *He also spearheaded the educational portal Alzheimer's Universe (www.AlzU.org).*

Discoveries about the prevention and medical management of dementia are emerging so quickly that we both marveled how much had changed since we talked for the first edition of this book.

Some families hear a certain drug can fix this. Or they've read on the Internet that something like coconut oil can cure Alzheimer's, and they come to me to find out how much to take. At the opposite extreme, others come to me frozen with fear. They haven't been able to figure out what they can or should be doing therapeutically after getting an Alzheimer's diagnosis. It can be hard for everyone to know what's realistic, what to try.

I always start by saying, "Let's take 10 steps back." Are you certain your loved one has Alzheimer's (and not another condition)? What stage? Does he or she also have other diseases? What are current lifestyle habits? I try to develop a broad management plan for that individual. It's not about one thing.

Unfortunately, Alzheimer's treatment isn't one-size-fits-all. It's not yet as straightforward as, say, treating high blood pressure. We can't just say, "Eat less salt." With Alzheimer's, there are more variables, there's more to explain—and the stress is higher for the caregiver, so there's a lot to talk about.

The science is changing so fast. We're at the point where we know enough to say everyone can and should be using dietary strategies as part of a prevention or treatment plan for Alzheimer's or memory loss in general.

The big "but": How well an individual responds to treatments boils down to genetics. You can throw the kitchen sink at someone and see little effect. You might say, "My Grandpa did everything right, he worked in the fields, he never smoked or drank, and he still got sick." I understand that frustration. What we don't know is, if he had done everything wrong, might he have gotten sick five or 10 years sooner?

Different people will respond to therapies in different ways, depending on their genes. We know some people are clearly helped by diet and lifestyle changes. We just don't know yet who benefits most. There's also a lot of complexity in the dose, the duration, how you take it, when you take it—a lot of unknowns.

The future for Alzheimer's prevention and management lies in precision medicine—evaluating, tracking, and refining what an individual needs based on their unique profile. Mr. Smith may need one kind of treatment, and Mrs. Jones something else.

In our clinic, we evaluate what I call the ABCs of Alzheimer's prevention and management: A is anthropometrics (your body composition, or fat and muscle distribution). B is blood biomarkers (things like metabolism, blood sugar, cholesterol, inflammation, other nutritional markers, genetics). C is cognitive function (using computer-based cognition tests). We look at the person's baseline for all three and re-evaluate every six months to see how their trajectories change.

Our patient histories also ask very detailed questions because we're learning that early life can be super impactful. We look at where you're from, sleep habits, education (even things like test scores), whether you play a musical instrument, how you lower stress. All kinds of surprising details can have a protective or harmful effect on brain health over time. I mention this to demonstrate how individualized care needs can be.

The good news is that there are interventions we can suggest to anyone now that have little downside. The risk is low, and the potential for benefit is moderate or high.

A lot of this is hot-off-the-presses data. Barely a decade ago, there was little high-quality, scientific evidence that once you developed Alzheimer's, you could change the progression by what you eat. But there's been an explosion in rigorous data, something new literally every week or month. What was once a very hazy field is now full of findings that can be put into clinical practice.

For example, the MIND Diet (a combination of the Mediterranean and DASH diets that emphasizes 10 brain-healthy food groups) has been shown to offer a 53 percent risk reduction for dementia. Sounds crazy? It makes sense to me—and we're now trying to fine-tune these "greatest hits" of dietary patterns. An ongoing randomized study comparing brain-healthy diets and the Western diet, for example, is taking place from 2018 to 2023, with results following 2 to 5 years later. But do we have to wait for the results? No. We have a ton of evidence that both the Mediterranean diet and the MIND diet are safe and brain-healthy.

No magic bullets: Try not to over-focus on berries, cocoa powder, or some other isolated nutrient. It's likely a combination of factors within a healthy diet is what makes a difference in the brain. And the healthy diet seems to work in combination with other lifestyle effects, as well as your genes.

Some of the risk-reducing effects from dietary changes are as large or larger than you see with the current FDA-approved medications for Alzheimer's. But there are no guarantees. Just as no single risk factor (not even old age or genetic predisposition) means an individual is necessarily going to develop Alzheimer's, no protective or risk-reducing factor (not even a brain-healthy diet) can guarantee that someone won't develop the disease. It's about reducing risk and slowing progression.

Notice I talk about prevention and treatment together. Although there are some differences, many of the same interventions apply. So if you're the caregiver of someone with Alzheimer's, you're smart to adopt "treatments" yourself, because you're already at higher risk of developing the disease. And most of these practices can, coincidentally, lower the risk of other chronic diseases, like heart disease and diabetes.

My top 6 lifestyle strategies for preventing and treating Alzheimer's: This list might sound like you've heard it all before. But there's solid evidence that steps like these have the lowest risk and the highest potential benefits:

1. A brain-healthy diet. In a nutshell, it's low-carb, antioxidant-rich, lower-saturated fat, low-glycemic index, and high in omega-3 fatty acids (especially DHA and EPA). Basically that means: Eat less bread and sugar (which raise blood sugar quickly) and more carbs from fruits, vegetables, and whole grains. Have fewer saturated fats (like butter and cream) and more brain-protective fats (such as avocado, olive oil, or omega-3 fatty acids in fish). Eat more lean protein (like fish or chicken). As or more important than the amount of fat you eat is where it comes from: Choose milk, yogurt, cheese, and beef from grass-fed sources, which are higher in omega-3 fatty acids.

2. Regular physical exercise. Several recent studies have shown the positive benefits of physical activity (from regular exercise to household chores) in possibly reducing the risk of Alzheimer's and mental decline, even in people older than 80. Recent data has shown that regular exercise maintains heart function, and that alone relates to a larger brain volume.

More recently, scientists have discovered that exercise reduces the pathologic protein in the Alzheimer's brain called amyloid (or beta-amyloid protein). Most physicians tend to believe that more exercise is better. For example, walking just 20-30 minutes a day, a few times a week, can make a big difference, yet 30-45 minutes several times a week may help even more. As long as it's been approved by the treating physician, exercise is generally among the most important things a person can do to preserve memory.

3. Cognitively-stimulating activity. This could be social connections, an adult-education class, or playing an instrument. Music activities are especially brain-stimulating. People who have engaged in lifelong musical activities have been found to have added protection against cognitive decline and memory loss.

4. Low to moderate alcohol consumption. It's okay for you and your loved one with Alzheimer's to have a small glass of wine with dinner, as long as it doesn't seem to affect thinking skills or behavior. There's no evidence that drinking helps with memory loss, though some research shows that one serving for women or one to two for men per day—especially red wine—may minimize the likelihood of developing Alzheimer's. Always drink with meals and not within 4 hours of bedtime.

5. *Social engagement*. Make time for supportive friends and family, even if it's just a shared cup of coffee with a neighbor or staying in your book club while caregiving. Think of it as buying time, not wasting time. Staying active and engaged in life, through adult-education classes, hobbies, and other social activities may synergize with a brain-healthy diet and exercise program to provide additional benefits.

6. *Adequate high-quality sleep*. Sleep is the newest frontier when it comes to Alzheimer's prevention and management. Believe it or not, you can do all the exercise in the world to loosen the bad amyloid protein in the brain, but if you don't sleep well, the amyloid can't be disposed of. During deepest sleep, the glymphatic system (a recently discovered plumbing system for disposing of toxins) "takes out the trash" in the brain. Without adequate sleep, the brain can't detoxify. We've also learned that low REM sleep (the "dream" sleep that happens about 90 minutes after you fall asleep) may be a risk factor for Alzheimer's.

Rome wasn't built in a day. Start by making the small changes that feel most do-able. Add a morning walk to your routine with your loved one. Have berries with your morning cereal. Find an activity that gets you both out and exposed to others. Try wearing a tracking device; there's evidence that using one to track things like steps and sleep motivates people to increase their brain-healthy lifestyle patterns.

Some people already diagnosed with Alzheimer's would benefit from what I call the "early bird special" a few times a week— dining early and waiting at least 12 hours between dinner and breakfast. There's mostly animal evidence so far, but fasting can bring about a very mild state of ketosis, where brain/body metabolism produces substances called ketone bodies. Ketone bodies may have a protective effect on brain cells and also may improve memory in people with mild cognitive impairment or Alzheimer's. (People with diabetes should avoid this, as well as very low-carb diets, due to health risks.)

What about Alzheimer's drugs? Medications may help some people more than others. Some doctors find them marginally effective, while others see greater success. Again, it's not an across-the-board thing. There are probably genetic influences we don't know yet. There are now drugs available that have been proven to work across all of the stages of Alzheimer's disease.

There's now strong scientific evidence to support use of these drugs over a few years. In my clinical practice, I've found that roughly 30-40 percent of patients stabilize at least for the short-term on these drugs, 30 percent improve, and 30 percent will continue to decline no matter what we try.

In addition to improving activities of daily living, like participating in conversations and feeding oneself, I believe that these medications can take the edge off negative behaviors, like agitation and aggression—and that can help ease the burden of the disease on both the patient and his or her entire family

To boost the clinical benefit, I typically recommend folic acid supplementation to patients on cholinesterase inhibitors (Aricept, Exelon patch). Or you can eat more dark leafy greens and citrus to get this.

Unfortunately, it doesn't help that for now you can see ten different doctors and get eight different opinions. Some doctors say, "Well that study shows therapy x may only work in 40 percent of patients. In six out of ten it won't, what a waste!" But if four in ten benefit, that's higher than zero in ten.

I would add: Consider participating in a clinical trial. I recommend this to people who are diagnosed with mild cognitive impairment due to Alzheimer's or mild/early-stage Alzheimer's (and their families) not just to "advance science" for the greater good, although that's great. It's to get state-of-the-art care that can be as much a pillar of a treatment plan as medications, vitamin supplements, and lifestyle approaches.

You get access to medications that won't be in the market for years. (Even if you get a placebo, after an initial period, most participants are offered a chance to try the drug.) After decades of failures, today we have enough data and a base of knowledge to set up trials in a different way, such as using biomarkers and genetics to qualify the right people, for example, to the point where it's very exciting.

We all—patients, caregivers, and physicians alike—need to balance expectations with realism. Some people expect the disease to retreat. We know that's not realistic. The goal is to slow progression, to stabilize the disease for as long as possible (or to delay the onset of Alzheimer's disease). If you stabilize someone for six months or a year, or if you delay getting it yourself for a decade, that's a win!

o o o

Leeza Gibbons: In the Meantime, Please Don't Harm Yourself

The TV personality and Alzheimer's activist wants you to do one thing today: Move yourself up to the top of your to-do list.

The oversize kitchen of her airy Beverly Hills home shrinks to cozy, coffee-klatch familiarity as Leeza Gibbons leafs through a family photo album. She laughs about a leopard-print bikini that was a favorite of her beautiful mother—"a cross between Jackie Onassis, Cher, and June Cleaver"—who had insisted on packing it for her move to a care facility, "just in case." And Gibbons tears up as she recounts the day that "sassy, sexy," and beloved woman no longer recognized her.

Hearing her authentic Alzheimer's tales, it's easy to forget that Gibbons is a media personality with a star on the Hollywood Walk of Fame, a face you first met in your own kitchen, on the TV screen when she was an "Entertainment Tonight" co-host and, later, host of her own talk show, "Leeza."

"Don't hide it. Make it count," Gloria Jean Dyson Gibbons had urged her journalist daughter upon learning that she had the same disease that had killed her own mother. So Leeza, co-host of the daily syndicated TV news show "America Now" and "My Generation" on PBS (for which she won an Emmy in 2013) and the 2015 "Celebrity Apprentice" winner, did. She created the nonprofit Leeza Gibbons Memory Foundation in 2002. Its centerpiece: Leeza's Care Connection, community support and education centers for caregivers. In addition to hosting fundraisers such as the Dare2Care gala, she wrote Take Your Own Oxygen First: Protecting Your Health and Happiness While Caring for a Loved One With Memory Loss.

TV host Larry King describes the Alzheimer's activist and caregiver advocate in terms anyone dealing with the disease would do well to emulate: "For Leeza, there is only one way to move, and that is forward."

Mom first began showing symptoms of the disease when she was in her late 50s. One day she confessed to my dad that she'd paid the same household bill three times. After that, we all started noticing things about her behavior that just "weren't Mom."

She started using profanity after never having cursed a day in her life. She repeated herself. She made paranoid, outlandish accusations to my dad, saying that he'd never loved her and was going to kill her. (He adored her.)

We thought maybe it was alcoholism, though she was just a social drinker. We were in a state of denial. Maybe it was a combination of Dad covering up for her behavior and our not really understanding what was wrong. I guess none of us wanted to believe that our wonderful mother might have such a terrible illness.

I wish I'd known what a marathon this is. Battling Alzheimer's disease is an endurance race, the likes of which I could never have imagined. My mom was diagnosed young, at 63. She died young, at 72. In between, as Nancy Reagan used to say, it really was the "longest goodbye."

This thief of life, thief of memories, isn't content to take just the diagnosed individual—it wants the whole family. It can suck you into a deep, dark hole unless you take steps to bolster yourself physically, spiritually, and emotionally. I was distressed to learn that stress-related disorders can take 10 years off a caregiver's life, and that caregivers often experience so many stress-related challenges that they get sick and die before the one they're caring for.

Compassion fatigue is a very real syndrome, and it can take down the best. At Leeza's Care Connection, we say you should "take your oxygen first," meaning: Nourish yourself before you take care of anyone else. Keep your body strong. Give your soul some strength, too. Take a break. Forgive yourself, forgive others. Do those things first.

The ultimate loving and selfless act is to first love yourself enough to care for yourself. Think of it as an investment that will allow you to love and support the person who's sick. When I felt my reserves were depleting, I'd remind myself to stop achieving and start receiving.

The caregiving challenge became hardest for my father, as my mother's disease progressed. I worried about Dad when Mom could no longer express her appreciation or her love but instead lashed out with anger at almost everything. I worried about Dad when Mom would turn around in the kitchen with a spatula in her hand and start swinging at him. I worried about Dad every night when he would go to his room and close the door, knowing we were losing him along with my mother. They were married for 55 years, but ten of them were stolen by Alzheimer's disease.

If you tore a page from my diary from this period, it would be shocking. Every day I felt frustrated by some new change or behavior. I'd lose my temper. I'd make mistakes. I'd feel overwhelmed. I was snapping at my kids, getting distracted by everything. I began to wonder what on earth had happened to the old me and if she was ever going to return.

Nobody is a natural-born Florence Nightingale or Mother Teresa all the time. I know I wasn't. I'd look at other people and think they had so much wisdom and patience, and then there was me. I was so not those things! But I learned that no one takes their first step on this path with all the answers. Heck, I didn't even know most of the questions.

Here's the thing: Being a caregiver allows you to either come face-to-face with the truth that we are all perfectly imperfect, facing vulnerabilities that are better handled with support—OR you can use your situation as a reason to prove that life isn't fair, that no one understands, and that you have to do everything yourself.

Guilt can become a constant companion. I've never met a caregiver who didn't feel some of it. So recognize it and let it go. When I was with my mom, I felt guilty that I wasn't going to see her enough. When I was away from her, I felt guilty for not being there. If I was out laughing and enjoying my life, I'd feel guilty because I knew Mom couldn't enjoy her life. If my sister was spending more time with Mom, I'd feel guilty. I'd even feel guilty because I was healthy and she was sick!

It helped me to repeat to myself a little mantra I made up: "I love my mother. I'm doing the best I can."

More of my favorite self-care advice:

- When someone asks if you need anything, get comfortable saying yes—and provide a list they can choose from. Don't be afraid to let people know what's helpful to you.

- **Break your responsibilities into bite-sized chunks**. Make lists: What do I have to do just today, just this week. Promise me you'll put yourself high on those lists, each day, by doing small things that cover the basics of being good to yourself physically and emotionally.

- **Don't ignore sleep**. (Remember sleep?!) Not getting enough of it undermines everything. Try a bedtime ritual like tea or a short walk to signal it's time to let it go. If your loved one keeps you up more than three times a week, keep a notebook of what's going on, so you can look for patterns and bring this information to the doctor.

- **Get empowered by those who have been through it before**. Maybe your "team" won't be made up of the usual suspects. Look for people who have patience, who allow you to be completely honest, who have been there, too.

- **Become an optimist**. I know it sounds counterintuitive, because you hear so much that may seem hopeless. But the lens through which you create your world affects everything. Those glass-is-half-full people really have an advantage. Know that you can do it. Thousands of people have.

- **This one's from my Dad. He should know**: "Worrying about what will decline next or wishing you could recapture something from the past will only prevent you from being in the present moment. As flawed and difficult as it may be, that's where life is."

o o o

"If you've seen one family facing Alzheimer's...well, you've seen one family facing Alzheimer's."

—Lisa P. Gwyther, director of the Duke Family Support Program

2: YOUR PERSONAL STORY

Situational advice, because no two dementia-care paths are the same

There's no single "caregiver journey."

Dementia strikes our partners, parents, in-laws, grandparents, dear friends, colleagues. The person may live with you, down the block, across town, or across the country. You may be geographically and emotionally close to the person with dementia, or not so much. While this book is primarily written for family caregivers, its insights and advice apply to anyone who wants to learn more, including those with more formal care relationships, like aides, social workers, and elder companions.

We all get into this in different ways. We help in different ways. We're all affected in different ways.

Worth noting: We're not even all grappling with the exact same disease. Alzheimer's disease is a specific form of dementia. It's in the title of this book because it accounts for the most cases—and is the sixth leading cause of death in the U.S. But there are many other forms of dementia, which share many similarities despite their few big differences. Confusingly, these are sometimes all lumped together and referred to colloquially as "Alzheimer's" or as "dementia," partly for convenience sake and partly because most people never get a precise diagnosis.

To muddle things still more, it's now known to be quite common for someone to have more than one neurocognitive disorder at the same time.

One study of autopsied brains found that the majority of people with dementia over 80 had this "mixed dementia" (for example, Alzheimer's plus vascular dementia). The specific mix of behaviors and cognitive changes you see depend on which brain changes are at work.

Along with how a person thinks and behaves, personality is also affected, sometimes in unpredictable ways. For your particular loved one, his or her core essence may always seem the same. More typically, though, noticeable changes in personality emerge early on. Over time, temperament and character can seem to alter dramatically. Having an awareness of which type of dementia personality you seem to be dealing with can also inform your care.

In light of these many variations, this chapter highlights special information to help you make the most of your particular dementia-care experience. It covers:

1. Your unique care role

2. The different types of dementia (good to know even if you aren't sure which you're facing)

3. Possible ways dementia re-shapes personalities

o o o

WHAT'S YOUR CARE ROLE?

A single case of dementia ripples outward. All of the affected person's relationships are touched, shaping our priorities, worries, and needs in differing ways, depending on where we stand.

Here, some critical do's and don'ts for specific dementia-care situations:

FOR SPOUSES

Yours is the most layered, wrenching, and demanding journey. The emotional changes (and yes, losses) are incalculable. Life partners set out facing this challenge as they have others, together. The regressive nature of dementia, however, by definition brings imbalance. One partner gradually diminishes and becomes more dependent on the other. The nature of even the most loving partnership is stressed. For all these reasons, spousal caregivers also face the greatest physical risks to heart health, brain health, and the immune system of any group of caregivers.

Do this:

Look for ways to balance hanging onto your old life while accepting the new. Grief, anger, guilt, fear, loneliness, and other hard emotions are virtually unavoidable. To stay productive in the present, though, many spouses facing a partner's dementia talk of the need to loosen a long-held vision of the marriage and to come to a level of acceptance with the new reality. They say an open-eyed honesty can be the best way to protectively support your partner while also protectively moving forward yourself. It's important to keep moving forward as a curious, creative, caring person for both your sakes. Supportive routes that others have used to find this delicate balance include mindfulness, prayer, talk therapy, and support groups designed for spousal caregivers.

Use your closeness to its maximum advantage. People with dementia tend to mirror the moods of those around them. Because many longtime partners are deeply in tune with each other from years of practice in good health, this tendency can be magnified.

If you can project patience, calm, reassurance, and kindness, in quantities greater than what you might be feeling, you possess an important tool for helping your mate stay on an even keel. Conversely, a spouse's irritation, anger, criticism, and exasperation can intensify negative behaviors. Things that help: Keep up old favorite shared activities and social connections as long as you reasonably can.

Find one or more people in whom you can confide. At times you're apt to feel frustrated, isolated, even abandoned. Not that your partner can help it, but he or she will be less able to provide the emotional support you're used to and need more than ever. Your social life can wither as you put your energies elsewhere. Old friends may surprise you by backing away out of discomfort or fear. Reach out to those you trust and can be candid with, even if it's just one or two people, and even if it feels a bit traitorous to confide openly outside your union.

Clarify what you expect from adult children. Many conflicts can be prevented through open conversation early in the disease, ideally when the parent with dementia can weigh in on preferences and wishes. The biggest mistake most families wait is ignoring the "elephant in the room"—cognitive impairment—for too long, postponing or avoiding the chance to talk about these tough issues. It can be especially useful to look forward together when your family involves such potential complications as stepchildren, a history of family problems, a family-owned business, or big geographic distances.

Develop a care circle. Every month, think of one resource you might add, from finding a day program to enlisting a neighbor to run an errand. Include your needs in the definition of that circle (in-home haircuts? finding a way to continue with your treasured book club?) because resisting isolation is a very real challenge for spouses. The mere exercise of thinking through possible options will move you toward using more of them.

Explore ways to connect with others who are in your same boat. Along with local dementia support groups for couples or spouses available through some medical centers and dementia groups, look into established groups like the Well Spouse Association or the Alzheimer's Association's spousal forum.

Avoid this:

Don't hide behind a façade. That's the vision of your marriage you present to the outside world, the one where everything's hunky-dory, you're in it together, and you don't let others in 'til death do you part. What's noble and admirable in healthy times becomes isolating and untenable by later-stage dementia. Nobody can be what you are to your partner, nobody can manage things just as well as you. Push past that. Marriage is sacred, but Alzheimer's care takes a village.

Don't postpone planning future financial and household management. Locate or obtain passwords and other account-access information. Get your name added to accounts. Pay special attention to possible Veteran's benefits (including knowing where the necessary records to apply may be found), pensions, trusts, and other benefits. Together or separately you may want to consult an eldercare attorney to guide you.

Don't read apathy, resistance, or irritation as reasons to get mad or give up. One of the main offsets to caregiving stress for spouses is feeling their help is noticed and recognized, research by University of Buffalo psychologist Michael Poulin showed in 2017. With Alzheimer's, this appreciation is in short supply. Someone with dementia often becomes self-absorbed and incapable of expressing gratitude. That's an inevitable byproduct of the disease—but hard to take. Knowing to expect it can ease the sting.

Don't brush off others' concerns about you. Spouses tend to cling most tightly to dangerous "always" and "never" vows. ("I'll always look after you." "I'll never put you in a home.") With Alzheimer's, all bets are off and vows sometimes have necessary limits. Many spouses report a huge improvement in their relationship and well-being once that partner is in an assisted living setting, absent the daily grind of struggling to care for a partner with significant dementia. It's possible to be able to care better and enjoy one another more, when you're not doing the 365/24/7 care.

Please keep reading: Much of the advice in the next section can also apply to you; in particular, it's good to be aware of the signs of depression and burnout listed.

FOR OTHER LIVE-IN CAREGIVERS (ADULT CHILD, GRANDCHILD, OTHER RELATIVE, FRIEND)

Among the benefits of having someone with dementia live with you: the satisfaction that you're making a tremendous difference, firsthand enjoyment of waning good moments, and an immediate grasp on what's needed. Your burden, on the other hand, is the grinding relentlessness of it all.

Do this:

Set boundaries to protect the other key relationships in your life. Watch out for "care creep" as needs increase. Dementia care can be a long haul.

You simply can't put the rest of your life on hold for the duration—much less expect your spouse/partner and children to do the same. It's understandable to feel you "owe" a parent or other loved one who did so much for you. But that giving can't come at the expense of those who enrich your life (and vice versa) in so many ways right here and now. Not prioritizing them is a sure path to making nobody very happy, you included.

Prioritize your own health and sanity. You won't find advice here about making time for bubble baths and spa escapes. (Ha, as if!) I'm a firm believer, though, that at minimum we all can, and deserve, to make smarter eating choices, sleep 7 or 8 hours as best we can, move our bodies, and have outlets that let us release some stress. If caregiving isn't allowing you to do those basic life requirements, you can bet resentment, depression, and health consequences will follow.

Shore up access that will help you protect assets. Key things you (or someone else in the care circle) need, at minimum: Power of attorney for finances, HIPAA access/clearance, power of attorney for health care, critical passwords or access codes, and an understanding of the basic financial picture. In dementia's mild stage (and sometimes moderate stage), your loved one will still have good-enough days to weigh in on preferences for these decisions.

Reach out to others who can extend your care capacity. Don't only connect when you need something. Update relatives and friends generally on a regular basis; they'll be more invested in helping when you need it.

Be explicit. Consider outsourcing the ask, too: If making requests is awkward for you or your relationship isn't great, try enlisting a neutral third party to nudge a sibling or adult child into doing something you need help with. It may be harder for them to say "no" to that person, and it underscores the importance of the need.

Arrange for all bills, calls, and correspondence to be routed through you (or one designated person). What sounds paternalistic is an often-overlooked safety measure. Judgment and decision-making abilities erode early and this step can help you avoid everything from missed bills or forgotten messages to financial scams and unnecessary charges. Try to monitor credit cards as soon as you suspect cognitive issues; even in the least likely people, problems with their use can show up.

Spread the burden of care early. Given that you're likely facing a long journey, it pays to set healthy patterns for everyone right away. Get relatives to have a stake in helping even before the needs rack up. Maintain an ongoing master list of responsibilities—then brainstorm what can be outsourced. Tap not just family but community resources (home delivery, transportation, meals, day services).

Try drawing a "CareMap" to visualize who's out there to help. It's as simple as literally doodling labeled stick figures (or x's and o's) representing everyone in your network: family, friends, services, your loved one's doctors and friends, and those who care for and support YOU. Then draw lines or circles that show how they're connected to you and to the person with dementia. This picture provides a quick glance at which needs are being met and unmet, who may be under-used or overlooked, and how everyone communicates with you and one another. It can also help you spark ideas for how this "ecosystem" might change over time. (For examples, see "Atlas of Caregiving" in Resources.)

Dementia-proof your home. Many safety measures are basic "universal design" principles that can benefit all of us as we get older. They don't have to look unattractive. Best improvements: shower grab bars and a sturdy in-shower seat, a taller-than-usual commode, and non-slippery surfaces (especially in showers and bathrooms). Also remove scatter rugs that can be tripped on, reduce clutter where important papers and items can get placed and lost, and add nightlights along the path to bathrooms.

Try to bend your habits into patterns that match what's easier for the person you're helping. Consistent sequences of events help make life predictable, and therefore manageable, as dementia erodes your loved one's sense of time.

Think ahead about your deal-breakers. The conditions under which home care would be impossible are different in every family. Few of us like to focus on this, but everyone has a limit. Common triggers for out-of-home care include when care needs exceed work obligations, incontinence, a physical mismatch (a smaller person can't help a larger one to the toilet, for example), aggression, wandering or other safety issues, privacy issues, and specialized health needs due to other conditions. Thinking about your limits ahead of time can ease guilt and help you plan ahead so you can act more quickly when needed. As these issues progress, they can be markers that prod you to research housing alternatives.

Avoid this:

Don't feel guilty if you can't devote every hour of every day to enriching the person's life while also offering basic care. People with Alzheimer's tend to do well when they have lots of sensory stimulation, activities, joy, and meaning. Creating such a life for them on top of managing everyday care basics, though? It's not for everyone. It's a lot of work to get someone to day services or to plan and execute special outings. It's time consuming even to plan in-home projects. Most family caregivers are also tending to jobs, children, partners, and/or their own personal lives and, contrary to a lot of dementia-care advice out there, can't devote 24/7 to the person with dementia. This is okay. Repeat: This is okay. If you do what you can to keep the person safe, secure, fed and healthy, you're doing a whole lot.

Don't expect others to "get" what your day-in day-out life is like. Sad but true: It's hard to appreciate unless you're in it. Inviting friends and family to spend 1:1 time with the person living with dementia gives them a window into your world. Nobody's a mind reader (and, to be honest, many of them don't like to think about it too much). You have to show and tell. And ask.

Don't get overly upset if others treat you as if you were invisible. The classic example: Family will call to ask how the person with dementia is doing but never ask how you're faring. Being taken for granted is a demoralizing byproduct of being a hands-on helper. Let go of looking for external applause and you'll let go of a lot of simmering resentment. (See also Chapter 4: "Personal and Family Stressors.")

Don't let disorganization add to your stress. Keep central files (both digital and for paper) for everything connected with dementia care: medical reports and instructions, insurance documents, resources, receipts, medication info, contact lists, and so on. You'll think you'll keep track of everything. But important details will get lost. I'm a big fan of baskets, the simplest catch-all organizer out there.

Don't ignore the signs of burnout and depression. What

might seem like "just helping Dad" or "doing what needs doing" can sneakily be killing you. Warning signs include a persistent feeling of anxiety, sadness, or hopelessness; frequent crying; deep fatigue; loss of interest in former activities or hobbies; difficulty concentrating or remembering details; lost appetite or overeating; poor sleep; thoughts of dying or suicide; and persistent aches or pains that don't ease up with treatment.

You don't have to experience all these signs to have depression, and their severity can shift. Consider them red flags that you, the helper, could use some help. Mention any you're experiencing to a doctor or make an appointment with a therapist. (Yes, absolutely tell your doctor you're actively caregiving even if you're not asked!) The majority of cases respond to treatment, says the National Institute of Mental Health, even the most severe.

FOR SUPPORTING CAREGIVERS

When you support the efforts of a hands-on parent, stepparent, or sibling (or other relative), you share similar concerns and feelings with them, if from a slightly different angle. The person with dementia will benefit tremendously from your understanding the condition and its effects, and from your involvement, whatever your degree of care collaboration.

A forewarning: The family relationships most torn apart by Alzheimer's are those between siblings, according to a 2017 Alzheimer's and Family Dynamics survey by the Alzheimer's Association. Almost two-thirds reported strife.

Do this:

Talk. We all assume things about everyone else, based on family history, gender roles, and other deep-groove factors. Assumptions lead to misunderstandings and hurt feelings. Though easier said than done, the more that can be communicated in a non-threatening, non-accusing way, the better. Keep the person you're helping at the center. Good rule of thumb: If you find yourself venting to a third party about something, you should probably be having the same conversation with the primary caregiver.

Learn enough about dementia care and the everyday routines to be able to step in as needed. Whether for an hour or overnight, every hands-on caregiver needs occasional relief. Some caregivers are reluctant to leave for a long period; you can always start small and build up.

Figure out which of your strengths you can apply. Sometimes they're obvious, like someone who works in the health care or insurance fields being able to act as the intermediary on those fronts.

Or maybe it's something about your personality; you may find that your patience makes you good at spending time with the person with dementia. Maybe your money or your time is your best contribution; for example, a flexible schedule that allows you to be a driver or handle medical appointments.

Keep repeating the magic words: "How can I help?" The degree of help will depend on your relationship and whether you live down the street, across town, or farther away. (See also the next section, "For Out-of-Town Caregivers.") Simply making yourself available is a huge first step. It's virtually impossible for the caregiving burden to be shared equally. Aim for a divide-and-conquer strategy, where everybody at least picks up some part (if not an equal one).

Give the primary caregiver the benefit of the doubt. You will see things done differently from how you'd do them. You may be brimming with suggestions for treatments based on what you read or hear. When it's a sibling or parent to whom you're used to saying what you think, you'll want to blurt it all out. Before you do, make an effort to understand the caregiver's point-of-view and stress level. Wrap your opinions in generosity and kindness, and back off unless you feel that someone is truly endangered.

Avoid this:

Don't put money at the heart of the situation. *How much of Dad's assets are paying for his own care? Why does she get her name on the checking account but not me?* How care is funded is an essential matter for families to agree on. Transparency and a voice for everyone go a long way toward keeping the peace. Still there may be grumbling. Try reducing some of the heat by keeping the focus on the person with dementia. If you're truly concerned about misuse of assets, and calm conversation with the primary caregiver goes nowhere, enlist a family mediator, attorney, or Adult Protective Services.

Don't live in the past. Try to shed ingrained old views of family members (untrustworthy kid brother, all-knowing mom, bossy sister). They get in the way of collaborating in the Now. As when you were kids, you won't agree on everything. You don't have to.

Instead, you have to find ways to get things done.

Don't take the main care provider for granted. Being the main contact person for someone with dementia is a lot, even when that person's doing well. Show thanks as best you can. Check in on how he or she is doing (asking not just how the person with Alzheimer's is). Offer up your time. Treat them. Just saying thanks is bigger than you know.

FOR OUT-OF-TOWN CAREGIVERS

You're not alone, not by a thousand miles. The current generations managing Alzheimer's are more scattered than any before. Whether you're monitoring a parent in the early stages of disease from afar or supporting a parent or sibling who is living with a person with dementia in another city, these added steps will help you make the most of your role:

If you're also the primary care contact, **Do this:**

Begin researching next-stage options early. During visits, use some of your time to stay one step ahead. Make proactive appointments to explore in-home supports, assisted living sites, hospice programs, whatever services the next stage might warrant. (You can do this without bringing the person with dementia.) Schedule doctor appointments for while you're there so you can establish relationships with providers and hear firsthand what's said.

Safeguard finances. Problems managing money are an early sign of dementia. Automate bill paying and get your name added to banking accounts if you can. Look for bills that are overdue or double-paid, large or multiple donations on bank statements, and lots of clutter that might be unopened bills. Pay special attention to how debit cards are used and consider switching to a pre-paid credit card or offering to close these accounts.

Consider working with a geriatric care manager if you can afford it. Also known as aging life care professionals, they provide holistic help ranging from assessments to planning, problem-solving, and advocacy—a worthwhile investment to spare yourself the stress and time of trying to manage everything yourself from far away. The Aging Life Care Association website has a directory.

If you're in more of a support role, **Do this:**

Provide regular relief for the close-by caregiver. Give your visits double purpose by spending time with the person with dementia while you're also giving the primary caregiver time off. Ideally, set up a predictable schedule of respite care (a weekend a month, two-week blocks once or twice a year, etc.) they can look forward to and count on. In between, offer emotional support by making yourself available to the primary caregiver as needed to talk—and then when you do, spend most of the time listening.

Take on care duties that don't require your physical presence. Examples: managing finances, handling insurance, coordinating services used, researching medical or housing options or Veterans benefits, providing financial support (especially things that make everyday life easier, like funding an elder companion or a lawn service).

Even small things, like helping to automate bills or stopping unnecessary catalogs and subscriptions, are huge burdens lifted from a live-in caregiver.

Realize that your perspective is especially valuable. Day-in, day-out caregivers often don't perceive changes in behavior or functioning as well because they make unconscious accommodations by small degrees. What you see may be upsetting for this reason (to you, the changes are more dramatic) but be persistent about mentioning your observations, especially if you can do so constructively. Have patience. It can take some time for the hands-on caregiver to see what you see.

Expect it to become harder to communicate from far away. Dementia will render faithful correspondents unable to write or type on a keyboard. Even the phone can become too frustrating to use. If you're braced for this loss you might feel less guilty about being unable to connect as regularly as you once did.

Avoid this:

Don't wait for a crisis to set up multiple communication channels. To stay in the loop, family members use everything from informal chat groups to standing times for videoconferences. Consider opening a rapport with local relatives, neighbors, and friends who can help act as eyes and ears on the ground. Know the names and numbers of key doctors, a local pharmacy, agencies or services used, insurance carriers, and utilities. Establish an emergency contact system too.

Don't be upset if your visits and attentions aren't

remembered or outwardly appreciated by the person with dementia. "Out of sight, out of mind" is as true for caregivers two blocks away as it is two states away. Although this hits you at your vulnerable spot (if you already feel guilty about not being available 24/7), remember that it's the result of a dementia-warped sense of time and memory. You know in your heart what you're doing!

Don't devote all your vacation and free time to visiting the person with dementia if you or your own family feels resentful about it. Obviously this is a deeply personal decision. Still, it's worth thinking hard about how much time you spend going to-and-fro because sustaining this over years can be rough. Providing respite to others is invaluable. There are plenty of other ways to help as well. It's a balance.

FOR CAREGIVERS OF SOMEONE IN A LONG-TERM CARE FACILITY

If your loved one is living in a residential setting, it's wise to still learn about dementia's effects, albeit with less emphasis on physical care and more about how to make the most of your time together and understand the needs of the moment. Like all caregivers, you're likely navigating difficult emotions and relationships with others who share an interest in the person with dementia. And you have an added layer of doing all this with (and sometimes in spite of) the facility.

Do this:

Make an effort to get to know, and thank, staff in order to gain better communication and better care. Pretty basic, but big. Learn and use aides' names. (Expect turnover. Learn new names.) Say thank you. Occasionally bring them food—not so much the sugary junk and bad pizza that everybody else brings but actual nourishing meals. That will stand out!

Use a memory book or poster to help staff know your loved one as a person. Some facilities, especially higher-end ones, do this routinely on move-in. If not, you can create your own makeshift version. Although aides, as much as they might care, are too busy to read a long biography, any kind of quick summary can help them to see the person beyond the "patient." Include primary relationships, past professions and interests, likes and dislikes.

Bring along some novelty and pleasure, to create an emotional state that will long outlast your visit. Some common mood lifters: music to share or an iPod and headphones with a special playlist, a game or old TV show to watch together a tablet, favorite treats (ice cream, a special pastry or comfort food), bringing your dog or cat for a short visit if it's okay with the facility, or stopping by with a young child (they're blissfully unselfconscious and pretty entertaining).

Raise any concerns that come up. Being an advocate for someone who can't fully engage on his or her own behalf might take you outside your comfort zone. Write down your questions and the answers you receive. Take detailed notes of any complaints, including specific times, circumstances, and the names of people involved. If you're told something can't be done due to rules or regulations, ask to see them. Some settings have a resident council where you can bring concerns. If you aren't satisfied with a response there or at care meetings, ask to speak to a higher-up administrator. Every facility also offers a state or local ombudsman to help resolve disputes. To find more help, look up The National Consumer Voice for Quality Long-term Care at theconsumervoice.com.

Avoid this:

Don't feel obligated to visit the person every single day. If you're able to and enjoy it, it's a win-win. If, however, it's a challenge to get there or if visits take a lot out of you, it's reasonable to be self-protective. (I've heard of doctors "prescribing" for their patients who are devoted but stressed caregivers to not make daily visits.) Similarly, don't feel you need to stay an entire day. The impact from half an hour may be the same because of changes in how time is perceived.

Don't take "I want to go home" at face value or as a rejection of the place. It's a hard-to-hear expression. "Home" might mean the person's most recent home, or any home in his or her past, even his or her room at the facility. Used by people with dementia, this common expression is less about a specific place to live than an idea of a place that's secure. Don't ignore it. Your loved one is expressing some kind of discomfort or insecurity—from fatigue ("I want to sleep now") to sadness ("Looking at these old photos is provoking").

First probe for more: "Tell me more about that." "What do you like about home?" If that's not helpful, try distraction, like moving to a different space or playing music. (See also in Chapter 3: "Help for Everyday Challenges: Confusing Communication.")

Don't be surprised to wrestle with guilt, sadness, and grief. They're all natural reactions to a disease that you can't change in any care setting. On the plus side—really do try to view it as a plus—not being responsible for 24/7 care gives you a chance to recharge, be present, and advocate for your loved one in ways that you may not otherwise have had the reserves for. For this reason, those who transition from being live-in to being out-of-home caregivers often find improvement in their connection to their loved one. They simply have more mental, physical, and emotional bandwidth.

o o o

ARE YOU DEALING WITH ALZHEIMER'S OR ANOTHER DEMENTIA?

Wait, what's the difference between Alzheimer's and dementia?

Dementia isn't a single disease but a term that describes a collection of behaviors and symptoms caused by brain changes that interfere with daily life. Alzheimer's is one of several different causes of dementia and by far the most common. Dementia is an umbrella term, meaning that if you have Alzheimer's, you also have dementia. But other things can cause dementia, too.

The term dementia itself was changed in the DSM-5 (*Diagnostic and Statistical Manual of Mental Disorders*, Fifth Edition), the 2013 update of the diagnostic manual used by mental health professionals. It's now referred to as *major neurocognitive disorder* and *mild neurocognitive disorder*. Most doctors and laypeople still use "dementia."

Does it matter what type of dementia you're dealing with?

Yes. But only to a certain extent. The #1 reason to have symptoms evaluated is to rule out the sometimes reversible causes of dementia symptoms. These can include medication interactions, brain tumor, normal pressure hydrocephalous (an abnormal accumulation of cerebral spinal fluid), thyroid problems, vitamin deficiencies, depression, and alcoholism.

There's yet no single test to diagnose the leading types of dementia. Confirmation with 100 percent certainty can only be made by examination of brain tissue after death. Nevertheless, doctors currently claim high accuracy rates in making a clinical diagnosis (95 percent accuracy for "probable Alzheimer's") through tools including taking an extensive history, tests of cognition and function, and process of elimination.

For non-reversible degenerative kinds of dementias, like Alzheimer's, the progression tends to be much the same, whatever the type. Important exception: Some behavior challenges and limitations are more common within particular types of dementia. That's useful to know, even if you aren't sure precisely which one your loved one has. More cases than previously thought are now considered to be "mixed dementia" or more than one kind.

My father-in-law's behavior so puzzled my husband and me that we were almost in denial about a connection to dementia, even though we both have professional experience in this area! He could carry on a long conversation about the Pittsburgh Pirates that involved pretty impressive working memory—their current ranking, which players were injured, whether the upcoming series was home or away.

One morning at breakfast, after half an hour of patter like that, he added without skipping a beat that he had a problem: "I'm getting married today and I don't have anything to wear." For the next few hours, he sat outside in his boxer shorts, waiting for an imagined suit to be delivered. As he was in his 90s at the time, we didn't pursue exhaustive testing, though a doctor noted that a prior MRI showed evidence of small strokes. Eventually it was clear his symptoms matched up to those of frontotemporal dementia, and having an understanding of it helped us be more empathetic and knowledgeable about how to respond—and a lot less freaked out.

Because every person is different—and it's often impossible to know exactly what's happening, biologically, inside a given brain—you may well encounter any of the situations described in this book.

Stages of Alzheimer's: Overview

You might be surprised to learn that there's no single definition of the "stages of Alzheimer's." Variously used staging approaches all reflect the fact that Alzheimer's is a degenerative disease (it gets gradually worse) that progresses along a spectrum.

Because you might encounter any of the following three most common ways of staging Alzheimer's dementia, I'm including all of them. The first one is the most useful to caregivers, I think, because of its practicality and ease of understanding. It's also fairly applicable to any type of progressive dementia.

1. Mild-Moderate-Severe dementia staging

Probably the most widely used staging system due to its simplicity, this approach refers to three main phases: mild (early), moderate (middle) and severe (advanced or late). Because they chart degeneration, they're sometimes further subdivided (early mild, mid-mild, late mild, early moderate, and so on).

A key insight: Skills and abilities are lost in the reverse order of which they're learned. So more advanced skills gained during adolescence, like paying bills, disappear well before basic skills mastered in infancy, like self-feeding.

Mild-stage Alzheimer's

The person can still manage basic self-care and communicate well, but memory changes are interfering with independent activities of daily living (IADLs), higher-order thinking skills, such as driving, shopping, preparing meals, and managing money or medications.

Think of mild-stage dementia as: Losing the skills that had been gained in the teenage years.

Someone with mild-stage Alzheimer's may:

- Repeat questions and comments
- Show poor judgment or an inability to plan or make decisions
- Get lost on familiar routes (walking or driving)
- Seem preoccupied or irritable, or show other personality changes
- Have trouble with basic finances, transportation, and medications.

Moderate-stage Alzheimer's

The person begins to have trouble with the so-called "activities of daily living" (ADLs), which are such basic skills as getting dressed, grooming, self-feeding, walking, and toileting.

Think of moderate-stage dementia as: Losing the skills that were gained during childhood.

Someone with moderate-stage Alzheimer's may:

- Remember the distant past better than more recent events
- Need help choosing clothes or dressing, brushing teeth, or bathing.
- Fidget restlessly, pace, wander away from home, shadow a caregiver
- Have delusions (fixed false beliefs), make false accusations
- Experience evening agitation known as sundowning

Severe-stage Alzheimer's

The person becomes unable to perform the activities of daily living without significant help. Basic life skills (speaking, sitting up, continence) are also affected.

Think of severe-stage dementia as: Losing essential skills that were gained during the first year or so of life.

Someone with severe-stage Alzheimer's may:

- Seem to lose all memory and live in a constant present

- Not talk intelligibly

- Not recognize even close family

- Have urinary and fecal incontinence

- Lose the ability to walk

Because people with Alzheimer's tend to have bad days and good days, it can sometimes be hard to tell where in the progression they are. If you look at the big picture, though, there is ongoing decline.

Another "stage" to know: End-stage Alzheimer's, also called "terminal dementia." This refers to the final days, weeks, to months of life. It's not identical to severe stage (for one thing it's almost always shorter) though they overlap. Because Alzheimer's is a terminal disease, the person will die from it in the absence of another health problem causing death first. (See Chapter 5: "End-of-Life Care.")

2. Diagnostic guidelines for Alzheimer's dementia and MCI

In 2011, classifying guidelines for clinicians were updated for the first time since 1984 following a two-year congress of leading researchers, sponsored by the National Institute on Aging and the Alzheimer's Association. The stages in these guidelines are as follows:

- ***Preclinical Alzheimer's***, also called pre-symptomatic: First defined in 2011, it's when changes are seen in biomarkers—for example, the nerve cells and blood—now that such biomarkers can be seen through brain imaging and other tests even when the person doesn't show behavioral or cognitive symptoms. This stage is currently of greatest value to researchers.

- *Mild cognitive impairment (MCI) due to Alzheimer's*: Mild changes in memory and thinking ability are noticeable to the person and to family and friends but don't interfere with the ability to carry out daily activities. Most, but not all, cases of MCI eventually develop into Alzheimer's.

- *Dementia due to Alzheimer's:* This is the stage most people think of as "Alzheimer's." Memory, thinking, and behavioral symptoms increasingly impair the person's ability to function in everyday life.

3. Seven stages of Alzheimer's (FAST Scale)

Developed by Dr. Barry Reisberg, this "global deterioration scale" (also called the FAST functional assessment staging tool) is a seven-stage assessment that's often used by researchers to evaluate patients. It's used less frequently by primary care doctors. The later stages include sub-stages that mark the loss of specific skills.

- *Stage 1:* No impairment; a normal person.

- *Stage 2:* Very mild cognitive decline (forgetfulness) that may or may not be normal aging.

- *Stage 3:* Mild cognitive decline: Memory problems obvious to others, trouble with complex tasks. Akin to mild cognitive impairment.

- *Stage 4:* Moderate cognitive decline: Increased trouble with IADLs, or instrumental activities of daily living (cooking, bill paying, cleaning, traveling). Mild-stage Alzheimer's.

- *Stage 5:* Moderately severe cognitive decline: Can't manage living independently without lots of help; needs help selecting clothes. Moderate-stage Alzheimer's.

- *Stage 6:* Severe cognitive decline: Moderately severe mid-stage Alzheimer's. 6a: Needs help dressing. 6b: Needs help bathing. 6c: Needs help with toileting. 6d: Increasing urinary incontinence. 6e: Increasing fecal incontinence.

- *Stage 7:* Very severe cognitive decline: Severe or late-stage Alzheimer's. 7a: Speaks only a few words. 7b: May say just one word a day. 7c: Can't walk. 7d: Can't sit up without assistance. 7e: Can't smile.

Other Common Types of Dementia

Besides Alzheimer's, other forms of degenerative dementia can cause similar symptoms and behaviors. Besides Alzheimer's, the most common forms are:

Vascular dementia (increasingly called vascular cognitive impairment)

- Second most common cause of dementia

- Caused by damage to the vessels that supply blood to the brain, often stroke ("post-stroke dementia") or small microstrokes the person may be unaware of but which deprive the brain of oxygen ("multi-infarct dementia")

- Similar in progression to Alzheimer's

- Often occurs along with other dementias, especially Alzheimer's

- Affects cognitive function (memory, reasoning, judgment, planning), disorientation (getting lost or confused in familiar places), and walk (shuffling steps)

- Appears in people with poor heart health histories, including high blood pressure, high cholesterol, smoking, diabetes

- It's also possible to have a stroke but not develop dementia, depending on the part of the brain affected and the amount of the person's cognitive reserve, which is the protective resilience that was built up over a lifetime of enrichment and other factors.

Lewy body dementia (LBD), also "dementia with Lewy bodies"

- Named for Lewy bodies, a type of abnormal brain protein deposit that alter brain chemistry

- Often starts with deterioration of thinking skills (memory, planning, understanding visual information) that seems like Alzheimer's but ability fluctuates

- Also causes visual hallucinations, sleep disturbances, problems with movement (tremors, slow gait, stiffness), and mood changes (depression and apathy to anxiety and agitation)

- A hallmark is REM sleep disorder, in which people physically act out their dreams

- Severely sensitive to some medication (antipsychotics and anticholinergics)

- Lewy bodies are also seen as an effect of the neurological disorder Parkinson's disease (Parkinson's dementia); sometimes Parkinson's diagnosis precedes LBD

Frontotemporal dementia (FTD)

- A broad term for dementias that strike the frontal and temporal lobes of the brain, causing them to shrink

- Still sometimes called Pick's disease, after the physician who first identified it

- Accounts for 10 percent to 20 percent of all dementia cases

- Often misdiagnosed as a psychiatric problem (depression, schizophrenia, alcoholism, even stress or menopause)

- Its most common form, behavior-variant frontotemporal dementia, often strikes in the 50s and 60s but can develop at any age

- First affects the parts of the brain where impulse control, judgment, and capacity for empathy reside

- Hallmark symptoms include dramatic personality changes, lack of concern or empathy for others, loss of good judgment, loss of shame and pride that can lead to socially inappropriate or compulsive behaviors, social withdrawal— and hauntingly, a lack of awareness about these changes

- Memory is often not affected; the person may recall things from both past and the immediate present pretty well

- Another type of FTD, primary progressive aphasia, tends to strike in midlife, affecting language skills. He or she finds it hard to write or speak even common words and becomes less able to read, follow a conversation, or talk

A way to help researchers learn more

This is a good place to mention that some families take solace in their loved one participating posthumously in dementia research, through brain donation. Unlike other kinds of organ donation, the purpose of brain donation is research only. Tissue is used in studies exploring the causes and treatment of Alzheimer's disease and other forms of dementia. As part of this, you typically receive a brain autopsy report, which is currently the only way to verify a specific kind of dementia diagnosis.

It can bring a sense of meaning to a terrible condition to be able to do something constructive at its end. Donating a brain doesn't delay funeral arrangements or interfere with an open-casket viewing.

But this is key: You'll need to plan ahead. If this option is of interest, contact one of the regional Alzheimer's Disease Centers (ADC) about obtaining a consent form and information about who to contact when the time comes. (See: Resources.)

o o o

WHAT TYPE OF PERSONALITY ARE YOU FACING?

Even before memory problems become exasperatingly obvious, family members often notice that a loved one seems "different" or "not himself." From early in the disease process, changes to the brain's systems of self-control and emotional regulation can result in noticeable alterations in personality. (Experts define personality as the sum of temperament, disposition, character, typical thought or activity patterns, and other traits that make an individual distinct.) In fact, these emotional and behavioral changes may be among the first effects of both Alzheimer's and frontotemporal dementia.

Often families see these changes but don't connect them to dementia. It's easy to believe a different problem is going on. A spouse might complain that a mate is growing rude or grumpy, for example—and the pair may bicker or grow apart. Adult children wonder if Mom's spaciness means she's drinking too much, or they take Dad's lack of interest in everything as a sign that he's bored by retirement. Actions that are actually the direct result of brain impairment are instead perceived as being done "on purpose."

None of these misperceptions are anyone's fault. Denial, confusion, and even sheer surprise about cognitive impairment are widespread and deep.

There's no single pattern of personality change in Alzheimer's. These four general patterns of change are most common:

1. Happy, in-the-moment

2. Depressed and/or anxious

3. Apathetic (unmotivated, uninterested, unemotional)

4. Paranoid, frightened, and angry

Consider them as four general "buckets" of demeanors and behaviors. There can be individual differences, and there can be some overlap between them. The type of dementia and the parts of the brain affected also influence personality changes.

The effect you see may be similar to the person's pre-dementia personality. In many instances, though, it feels like your loved one has had a personality transplant. Also, someone might start out one way and shift later. For example, depression and anxiety in the early stages of the disease may mellow into a disposition that's more content as awareness wanes.

It's useful to know that such patterns exist, because they can help you understand why your loved one is saying and doing the things that are so out of character. You can better prepare for what might be coming and find ways to manage things and make life more comfortable for the person and for you. And you'll be less likely to blame yourself for behaviors and incidents that don't really have anything to do with you personally.

Below you'll find detailed information about each of the four common patterns. Following these descriptions, the rest of the section offers advice on the specific ways these personalities manifest themselves.

o o o

Dementia Personality Pattern: Happy, In-the-Moment

My mother-in-law, Louie, was a classic Southern "steel magnolia." With her honeyed mid-Georgia accent, charm, and perfect manners, you might mistake her for just another pushover, a pretty flower. Once you got to know her, though, you saw that beneath this belle-veneer was a prickly lady of strong opinions and high expectations who wasn't afraid to pick a fight or hold a grudge. (I loved her!)

A funny thing happened as her dementia progressed, however. She became milder, mellower, easier-going. She seemed to let go of her need to control. When my son showed up with shaggy hair, there were no lectures about haircuts, just sweet-talk about how cute he was. When my daughters shifted from smocked dresses to short skirts, she applauded their taste instead of frowning. Once Waspily standoffish, she grew more huggy. More shockingly, she let other people clean up or do the dishes! She seemed happy just to...be.

That surprised me because Alzheimer's had turned my grandmother—who'd always had a softer, jollier personality than Louie—into a crotchety, sad shell by the end. My father, on the other hand, had lived his whole life happy-go-lucky, and (with an occasional few exceptions) had stayed that way throughout his dementia slide. —P.S.S.

What it looks like:

Sometimes called "pleasant dementia," this is perhaps the least problematic of personality changes you might see. The person tends to be docile and agreeable. They generally go along with suggestions. They're polite, expressing gratitude and thanks. They don't seem to fret about the past or what's next. Instead they take each moment as it comes. This ability to live in the moment seems to keep their mood relatively light, especially if they feel secure, loved, and well cared for.

"The burden of having to anticipate the future and prepare for it, and the burden of remembering things they don't like about the past, has been removed because of their cognitive impairments," says geriatric psychiatrist Kenneth Robbins. "They're now able to live in the moment and enjoy it."

Sometimes the person seems happier than she's ever been.

TRY this:

- **Do all you can to help the person have a stable existence, rich with security and routine**. This kind of care seems to help foster a calm, happy persona. (If you're not seeing this pattern, though, don't take it personally. Although quality of care influences behavior to some degree, it's not the whole story. Brain changes often trump good intentions and good care.)

- **Be generous with physical affection**. Hugs and hand-holding speak louder than words in creating security.

- **Continue to find stimulating activities and social outlets**. Because this personality type tends to be so agreeable and uncomplaining, it's easier to forget that they still have a need for stimulation and guidance.

To help you cope:

- **Allow yourself to experience the confusing stew of emotions these changes can bring**. I remember feeling a mix of relief (an easy personality is, well, easier than a querulous one), guilt (for feeling relief), sadness (because I missed the sharpness and the person I'd known), and a kind of bittersweet gratitude (because my mother-in-law was no longer aware of her deficits and seemed to be enjoying life as it was).

- **Take solace in the comparison that some researchers have drawn between pleasant dementia and that state of mind learned through meditation and mindfulness**. Its emphasis is on acceptance, letting go, being fully present. It's ironic that a loved one's reduced cognition should help show us the way: *What a beautiful sunset...I'm not mad at you anymore...no complaints here...why thank you...taking the scenic route...Who, me worry?*

o o o

Dementia Personality Pattern: Depressed and/or Anxious

Ron felt he was slipping up. At first he blamed new, complex office procedures, or maybe it was just a matter of getting older. It was becoming harder to concentrate at work. He missed a few deadlines. When he found it hard to track his business expenses, he quit turning in expense reports at all. ("It's not that much money," he told himself. But he never told his wife, Tracy.) Once he got confused in the Atlanta airport. For the life of him, he couldn't figure out where he was supposed to go. Eventually he tried to board the wrong flight. He missed the right one and might never have gotten home at all if he hadn't run into Bob from the team. That was embarrassing, but it sure was a lifesaver. After that, Ron avoided travel assignments.

He felt best in the evening, with a glass of bourbon in his hand and a sports show on TV. Then he could relax. When Tracy tried to talk to him about her concerns—she said he wasn't paying attention to her, harping about that fender bender again, nagging him to see the doctor about working too hard—he tuned her out.

Tracy, for her part, noticed Ron drinking more regularly. He seemed to be retreating inward, turning down social engagements and not going on as many business trips. She worried about how his job was going. She worried about his driving—two minor accidents and two tickets in the last six months. But when she tried to get him to talk about anything, he cut her off. "Do you think I'm a moron?" he'd snap. "Leave me alone!"

Then he'd start muttering about crazy drivers and inept colleagues in a fretful tone, and take another deep sip of bourbon.

What it looks like:

Depression and anxiety are especially common in the earlier stages of Alzheimer's disease, when the person still has enough insight intact to be aware that he's having increasing difficulty with his thinking skills. They may intensify as the disease progresses.

Imagine knowing something's wrong that you can't necessarily put your finger on, and worse, can't control. Nagging fears and unease begin to take over and leave you upset or down.

Feeling anxious about life (in general, or about specific incidents) causes the person to act irritable and fretful. He may express worry, fear, or dread, and have a hard time concentrating. Sleep may be affected. Physically, he may complain of headaches or stomachaches, and might tremble, sweat, or seem jumpy.

Associated behaviors include agitation, pacing, shadowing (closely following) a family member, hoarding, and avoiding be left alone.

Anxiety can slide into depression, or one can exist separate from the other, although their origins are similar. Depression can intensify memory problems.

Signs of depression are similar to those in people without dementia: changes in sleep (too much or too little), changes in appetite (eating too much or too little), loss of pleasure in things, a sense of hopelessness or worthlessness, sadness, agitation, and thoughts of death or suicide. (People with dementia who are depressed both tend to talk about suicide and follow through less often than the rest of the population.)

Almost three in four people with dementia are thought to have anxiety symptoms, and up to one in five people have an anxiety disorder. As many as half of people diagnosed with Alzheimer's show at least some signs of depression, and the depression can persist throughout the disease. (Depression is also a risk factor for developing Alzheimer's. People who struggled with untreated depression before dementia may continue to have it as a co-existing disease.)

TRY this:

- **Report symptoms to the doctor**. It's important to rule out other causes (such as a drug reaction or infection). Antidepressant medications are used to treat both anxiety and depression. Sometimes anti-anxiety medications are used on a short-term basis, but they tend to have side effects, including worsening memory and a greater risk of falls. That's why behavioral solutions tend to be the first course of action with anxiety.

- **Make sure the person engages with others**, since social isolation is known to feed anxiety and depression. In the early stages of dementia, a support group can provide both a social outlet and a safe place to talk about the stresses of adjusting to cognitive changes. Adult day programs are similarly helpful. Talk therapy can also help and is covered by most insurance plans.

- **Encourage exercise every day**. It can help both mood and any sleep problems the person with dementia may be having.

- **Minimize traumatic changes**. Moving, a hospitalization, or the loss of a consistent care partner can all intensify anxiety or depression. As much as is practical, it helps to keep to a supportive, consistent routine.

- **Step back to see if you notice patterns or triggers when behaviors worsen**. Each person tends to have his own triggers: bathing, talking about money, or being overwhelmed by too many people or frustrated by not being able to do a former task to one's former standards, for example. When you discover a trigger, try to take extra steps to remove it (no money talk, no big parties) or make it easier and less stressful to manage (introduce a different hobby, simplify bathing).

- **Help the person to feel busy and productive**. A sense of accomplishment, meaning, and purpose are critical to someone in the throes of anxiety or depression because of perceived losses (of ability, thinking skills, and the freedom of driving, among others). One French study exposed people with anxiety or depression and dementia to cooking, baking, and music. After four weeks, their symptoms decreased. If the person can no longer work, look for volunteer outlets where he or she can channel energy safely, rather than downshifting to doing nothing. Avoid taking over all chores; find ways the person can participate.

- **Set up a win-win environment, where challenges and frustrations are minimized**. Make it easy to find food and clothing and to navigate through the day. Help in an unobtrusive way.

To help you cope:

- **Realize that you'll need to play a fairly active role in managing this personality change**, so gear up with all the help and resources you can. Part of the challenge in this situation is that coping with feelings of anxiety or depression is hard for anyone (you may even be struggling with this yourself). But when you're cognitively impaired, you're virtually unable to drag yourself to a therapist, connect with a doctor, or confide in an old friend, and so on. Intervening and reassuring is an added burden on family caregivers, but your efforts can pay off in fewer disruptive behaviors down the road.

- **Expect mood swings or angry outbursts**—and when they happen, don't take them personally. Remind yourself of Duke's Family Support Program director Lisa Gwyther's adage: "It's the disease, not the person."

o o o

Dementia Personality Pattern: Apathetic (Unmotivated, Uninterested, Unemotional)

Gloria's frustrations with her husband's personality reached their peak the day their daughter brought the children over for Jack's birthday. Twins Ava and Aiden, 8, had made their "Gramps" a paper crown and helped to decorate his cake. They'd each picked out presents for him and couldn't wait to divulge their contents soon after they'd burst into the house.

"Whoa!" she said with a smile, bending down to hug each of them as they gibbered with excitement. Jack, who'd once loved spending hours teaching the kids how to tie nautical ropes or take care of his sailboat, never rose from his chair. He seemed to watch them all as if they were far, far away.

"Gramps! Gramps! Guess what we got you?!" Aiden shouted as he clambered onto his lap. "Hey! Gramps? Where are you going?"

To everyone's surprise, Jack had brushed off the hugs and hellos— and the grandchild on his lap. He stiffly rose from his recliner. Waving his hand back at the group, he shuffled out of the room. "I don't want any birthday."

The children just stared in astonishment.

What it looks like:

Also described as stunted emotions or a loss of motivation and interest in the world, this change tends to be readily recognized by family members early in the disease, though at first it might be mistaken for stubbornness, rudeness, laziness, or depression. The person may be passive and lethargic, withdrawing from former interests or showing little initiative in making plans or following through. Families often describe "something missing" from their loved one. It's especially noticeable in someone who once had a lively, active, leader-like personality.

"These are people who seem as though someone stuck a needle into their brain and removed any emotion," says geriatric psychiatrist Kenneth Robbins. "While they don't seem anxious, they've lost the capacity for joy."

Apathy in dementia is common, affecting 50 to 80 percent of cases. (In contrast, only 1 percent of healthy people suffer from apathy.)

Early on, apathy looks like this: Compensating for cognitive deficits takes a lot of attention and energy—and that creates an intense self-focus that can crowd out focus on other things, such as one's spouse or other family members, work, and outside interests. As the deficits progress, the affected person instinctively avoids what's frustrating or consuming and pares down attention to the most critical things: remembering where he put his glasses, tying his shoes. Extraneous noise, visitors, questions are tuned out.

Ultimately, changes to the part of the brain that handle initiation and planning—in the frontal lobes—may be responsible, scientists think. It's a kind of impairment in thinking skills known as executive function. These changes are separate from other cognitive decline and from how much emotional stress someone is under. Apathy tends to worsen as the disease progresses. What's more, those who show apathy tend to also show increased rates of cognitive decline and functional impairment, studies show.

Although some symptoms of apathy overlap with depression, they're considered distinct conditions. Someone with dementia who's depressed will also show strong emotions such as sadness, crying, hopelessness, or even suicidal thoughts. With apathy, there's just an emotional indifference.

TRY this:

- **Mention symptoms of apathy to the doctor**. A good psychiatric workup can be helpful in distinguishing apathy from depression. It's useful to know which you're dealing with, because someone with apathy is less likely to "snap out of it" with talk therapy and medication. Some people with apathy do improve on antidepressants, though, and some research has shown that Ritalin can boost energy and motivation.

- **Avoid nagging, cajoling, and accusing**. Someone who's apathetic can't help being the way they are.

- **Encourage physical activity**. It can make a critical difference to energy levels and mood.

- **Be prepared to provide extra support with functional, everyday tasks**, such as dressing, toileting, and feeding. Even for someone still capable, the wherewithal to begin these tasks or follow through has likely been lost. Step-by-step encouragement is key.

To help you cope:

- **Remind yourself that this is a personality pattern that can be hard to deal with**. Loving care, consistent routines, and encouragement can help move the person forward—but not always and not reliably. In other words, it IS the disease at work. It's not all up to you.

- **Arrange regular respite care for yourself**. An adult day center, an eldercare companion, or other sources of relief are important to your mental health. When dealing with an apathetic personality in someone with dementia, you tend to get even less back emotionally than you would in other situations. That can be incredibly depleting.

o o o

Dementia Personality Pattern: Paranoid, Frightened, and Angry

"Get rid of that one!" Astrid pointed a finger at her granddaughter, Beth-Ann, who was arranging some flowers across the bedroom, helping look after her during a college break. "She's the thief! She pretends she's messing with flowers, but the minute my back is turned she'll be in my jewelry case!"

"Gran, it's me, Beth-Ann. Nobody's stealing anything!"

"So where are my pearls?" she said, accusingly, reaching up to her bare throat.

"Gran, you're in bed. Why would you have pearls on?"

Astrid only glared and shouted, "Get out!"

Beth-Ann was shaken. Her mom and dad had warned her about these outbursts. Sometimes Astrid complained about men hiding under her bed at night and robbing her the minute she fell asleep. That's why she wasn't sleeping any more, she said. She muttered to herself a lot and was obsessed about the pearl necklace she used to wear. Once she lunged at a woman in a restaurant who was wearing a similar necklace and accused her of stealing it! When Beth-Ann's dad had tried to restrain her, she scratched at him. None of this behavior was anything like the sweet-natured Gran that Beth-Ann had grown up with.

What it looks like:

The paranoia of dementia can be baffling and deeply unnerving to families because it usually seems so out of character. In fact, when my father-in-law began showing such odd behaviors (grieving about his late wife's imagined affairs, telling detailed stories about them), my husband, at first, found himself wondering if they could possibly be true—in part because his dad seemed so much like himself in every other respect.

But paranoia and delusional upset are rooted in a strange kind of logic. Unable to comprehend what's going on in her own head and in the everyday world around him or her, someone with dementia feels out of control. Things don't make sense. Impaired thinking skills "fill in the gaps" to explain things with false beliefs (called delusions).

The granddaughter Astrid failed to remember is the thief of an imagined lost necklace. The aide who wants to help give a bath becomes a would-be rapist. Night shadows are goblins, birds talk to you, crime scenes on TV shows become a window on what's happening in the next room. An admired and loved wife who died and is terribly missed is cast as a wrongful party to explain such strong feelings.

As logic fails, the crippled mind of someone struggling with dementia might sense that everyone is out to harm her. These paranoid delusions are alternately frightening (which requires a lot of reassurance) or maddening (which can lead to anger and aggression).

The paranoid person with dementia may hallucinate, lash out physically, say outrageous and often cutting things, lie baldly, or show fear or mistrust.

No matter how much you try to reason or rationalize, these false thoughts can't be budged. Caregivers sometimes go to great lengths to "prove" fastidious accounting or the honesty and good record of an aide, but it's wasted effort. Logic can't cure delusions.

It's not clear how many people with dementia experience paranoia, but estimates hover around one in four. Paranoia, delusions, and inappropriate behaviors are common features of frontotemporal dementias. In dementia with Lewy bodies, hallucinations are common.

TRY this:

- **Listen empathetically and attentively, without really agreeing or disagreeing**. Use neutral phrases such as, "I'm sorry you feel that way," or "That must be upsetting."

- **Try deflecting the situation with a light touch if it works for the person**: "Oh Gran, nobody in the world could be as beautiful as you in those pearls. Let's put them on you and you can see. I'll get a mirror."

- **Sometimes it works to just wait out the moment and say nothing**. Or distract with a favorite activity, such as eating ice cream.

Tip: **"When my mom was saying crazy things, I'd make my cell phone ring and say, 'Oh, I have to take this call. Just a minute, Ma.' By the time my fake call was done, the** moment would often pass." —D.R.

- **If the person becomes physical and you feel endangered, talk to the doctor**. Paranoia is sometimes treated with antipsychotic medication, although this is considered a last-resort option. The FDA has warned that antipsychotics increase the risk of death in people with dementia. And although they often reduce delusions, they don't always eliminate them.

To help you cope:

Realize that delusions are almost never rooted in any kind of reality. It's not as if Astrid always secretly thought of her granddaughter as a sneaky type of girl and now is finally speaking the "truth." My father-in-law, who accused his wife of infidelity, didn't have such suspicions, or cause for such, in the whole of their marriage before the dementia. Instead, the person is reacting to something in the current reality: failure to recognize a granddaughter, a fear of being abandoned, loneliness.

Most delusions aren't rooted in anything you're doing, or not doing, in the present moment. It's not as if by caring harder or being more careful, the false thinking will disappear. The problem is rooted inside the brain.

Get a safety net of help and support for yourself. It can be incredibly draining and toxic to listen to false accusations or live in fear of being struck. Endlessly soothing and coaxing a paranoid, fearful person can feel like you're walking on eggshells. And that's stressful. You need regular respite care, along with someone you can vent to, whether a trusted friend or a paid talk therapist or counselor. Even though you may "know" this is the disease at work, living with it can eat away at you without the reinforcement and perspective-righting help of others.

o o o

"Realize it takes two to tango—or tangle."

—Teepa Snow, occupational therapist

3: HELP FOR EVERYDAY CHALLENGES

Why they happen, practical solutions to try

My friend Rachel called, obviously upset. She and her family had just taken their mom, Ann, out to brunch—and for most of the meal everyone was happy and relaxed, she said.

On her way to the restroom, though, Ann stopped at the next table to coo over a baby with bright copper ringlets. "Oh, I just love a baby with red hair! I was born a redhead," Rachel heard her say, patting the baby's head. "But when she hits the temper tantrum stage, look out!" Everyone laughed."

On the way back from the restroom, Ann again stopped at the baby's table—and repeated her earlier comment, word-for-word. This time the young couple just smiled politely. Rachel spirited her mom back to her seat.

"And then a few minutes later," Rachel told me, now getting teary, "Mom got out of her seat to go pat that baby's hair for a third time and told them the exact same story."

This time, the baby's parents seemed kind of freaked out by this strange woman who kept touching their baby. They pulled the baby away. Ann's family was stricken, too. They'd been noticing signs of forgetfulness but had never seen her do anything like that before.

"I apologized and hustled Mom out of the restaurant," Rachel said. "We were just finishing our coffee, but I was too embarrassed to stay. She was so mad, and kept saying, 'Why are you being so rude to this young couple? I don't want to leave!'

"I didn't know what to do."

Maybe you've already had an experience like that, or maybe it's farther down the road for you. Dementia places families in so many strange new situations of all kinds—and it's natural not to know how to react at first. Often the best response goes against your normal instincts. It's easy to lose your temper, for example, but getting angry only makes your loved one feel (and often act) worse.

This section highlights many of these problems, from the mildly annoying (like repeating stories and acting odd in public) to the downright scary (like aggression or wandering away). For each, I offer what I call the "Why-This, Try-This" approach. Knowing the reason for what seems like an "unreasonable" behavior can help you find more patience—and provide much-needed clues for what to do.

o o o

About the "Why-This, Try-This" Approach

Together, the words "why" and "try" can transform the way you live with the many vexing behaviors of dementia—and the effects they have on you.

"Why-This, Try-This" is, simply, a pathway to problem-solving. It has two parts:

1. WHY: Pause to consider why the person may be doing what he or she is doing. Alzheimer's behavior almost always has meaning. It's a reaction to a set of circumstances. So it's critical to ask yourself what is it about the disease, the person's feelings or background, or the situation that might be contributing to a given behavior. There may be one simple trigger or multiple things going on.

2. TRY: You can then use those clues to consider the different ways to try to change the situation. You can't change the fact of the disease itself. You can, however, use insights about it to alter most other variables—the environment, your reaction, what happens before and after, and so on. There's seldom one single "right" solution to a challenging behavior or situation. There are usually many different things you can try until you hit on one that works for you.

Once you develop the habit of thinking this way, you can get "unstuck" from unproductive responses that get you nowhere or make things worse. You can more quickly move to head off trouble.

Although you may feel like you're not an expert on dementia, you have the advantage of knowing your loved one and an awareness of the situation at hand. Add in some basic insights on dementia and the suggestions that follow, and you'll be following the "Why-This, Try-This" approach before you know it.

This chapter shows you how and takes out much of the daunting guesswork.

The "why" explanations presented are grounded in what we know about dementia—how it erodes memory and thinking skills, how personality can change, the hallmarks of how it typically manifests, stage by stage.

On top of this, Alzheimer's can magnify the ways that we all act when we're bored, frightened, upset, angry, or feeling insecure, and leave a person even less equipped to deal.

Along with the disease itself, the question "why" invites you to consider other possible factors in play. They, too, can provide clues to the best response. Play detective or reporter and consider the other 5 "W" questions:

- **WHO are you dealing with?** Even someone who seems changed by dementia retains many core preferences, motivations, and traits. This core, plus individual background and life story, health history, and current health status, can point you to answers or diversions.

- **WHAT else is going on that might be a trigger?** Is there something the person sees that you could remove from his line of vision? Is it noisy or quiet? Is it hot or cold? Did someone just say something that may have tripped a reaction? Is there a new caregiver around?

- **WHEN does it happen?** Every day? At the same time? Random times? Only when the sun does down? Or when he's tired or hungry? On hot days?

- **WHERE does it happen?** Out in public? While sitting in a particular chair or room? Indoors or outdoors?

All this information acts like a springboard to possible solutions. The "try" suggestions in this chapter are informed by the experiences of scores of clinicians and caregivers who have been down these paths before you. Over time, you might come up with your own solutions, too. As my father-in-law was fond of saying, even into his 96th year, "Whatever works!"

The beauty of "Why-This, Try-This" is that these insights help you take things less personally. They can leave you feeling a little less cross. They help you to not blame the person with dementia for behaviors he or she can't control. And they get you unstuck. With so many benefits backing two simple words, why not?

o o o

MEMORY CHALLENGES

About Memory Loss

Memory loss has become the poster symptom of Alzheimer's. That's because it's particularly upsetting to the person experiencing it and so frustrating for family members.

Other symptoms tend to appear earlier, including personality changes such as self-absorption and withdrawal, difficulty with money or math, getting lost, and trouble making plans or finding the right words. But because memory is so obvious and used in so many ways, it tends to be the first cognitive impairment symptom that families notice.

A quick overview of memory loss:

The cell damage of Alzheimer's disease (and most other forms of dementia) causes newer memories to erode first. Those that last longest tend to be very old memories (often of childhood) and emotionally rich memories (triggered by music or scent), possibly because these are stored in multiple areas of the brain.

Damage to the brain's active memory systems shows up early. One kind, short-term memory, is designed to help you function in everyday life. It allows you to recall who just said what in a conversation, why you walked into a room, what you ate for breakfast. Even in healthy people, short-term memories get crowded out by similar memories, so after a few days, it's natural to forget what you ate for breakfast three days earlier or what you wore last Saturday. It's also normal to be forgetful sometimes about what you just came into a room to do or where you parked your car. (This is often due to lack of attention.) A rule of thumb is that it's not too concerning if you remember that you've forgotten something, because that shows your brain is working on it. (*Darn, I left the grocery list at home!* Or, *What's that actor's name?*) Someone with dementia, however, doesn't realize he or she has forgotten. It becomes harder to form short-term memories at all, much less to retrieve them.

A type of short-term memory called working memory is also affected. That mental "scratch pad" is where we store bits of thoughts even more briefly, such as the phone number we just looked up to dial, numbers used in adding a column of figures, the time just viewed on the clock.

These scraps of information normally stay in our heads for a few seconds, allowing us to do something they're needed for, before vanishing so as not to clutter the brain with unnecessary information. With dementia, these working bits also can't be held. That makes it hard to follow directions, add numbers in a checkbook, or even put on a shirt.

Short-term memory is different from long-term memory, where events have more distinction and meaning. Long-term memories are often episodic (a story, an event) and tend to be reinforced by repetition. They're stored in multiple parts of the brain (unlike short-term memories) and can be held for decades, even a lifetime. Long-term memory can remain remarkably intact deep into dementia. A person who can't remember having just eaten or even his own daughter might recall the names of old teachers or tales from childhood, for example.

Many social skills and "muscle memory" (the ability to repeat a certain motion without consciously thinking about it) can also remain intact even though new memories can't be formed or retained. Someone with memory trouble may therefore seem perfectly capable, especially if he or she is actively trying to hide other limitations. It can be hardest to see a problem when the person is doing or saying rote things (doing dishes, exchanging social pleasantries) because these auto-pilot behaviors conceal some of the cognitive trouble.

Although memory loss plays a role in many different dementia behaviors, the following memory challenges are among those you're most likely to encounter.

o o o

Repeats the Same Questions or Comments Within Minutes (or Less)

When Rhonda's mother first began repeating herself, Rhonda chalked it up to "old age." She tried not to be impatient when, five minutes after telling her that her cousin Sue was visiting soon, she'd ask brightly, "When are we going to see Sue again?" Her two teenagers pointed out that their Mamaw often re-told the same story about something one of her beloved pets did over and over within an hour, using the exact same words and sentences each time. "The kids were very patient, but I'd lose my marbles and yell at her, which only hurt her feelings but didn't stop the repetition," Rhonda says.

Eventually, in the evenings, Mamaw would jump up from her chair every five minutes to ask, "Have the animals been fed?"

"She was like one of those German clocks where the wooden figure pops out—only not every hour—more like every two minutes," Rhonda says.

WHY it happens:

Often, a specific trigger is being pulled again and again: Glancing at the clock makes a woman wonder what time something is happening, for example. Or seeing a visiting grandchild begs the question, "So how old are you? Do you like school?" The questions and comments themselves are normal. It's the repeating that drives everyone bonkers.

Boredom or anxiety can aggravate repetition. Someone with dementia feels emotion continuously ("I don't want to be late!" or "It's my job to feed these pets!") even if she doesn't remember having just expressed the same idea.

The repetition can be a question, a comment, or an entire word-for-word anecdote.

TRY this:

At first...

- As much as you can, calmly and without comment, give the same answer. Keeping your patience is the biggest challenge.

- **Try not to point out, "You just said that" or "You just asked that!"** Erase phrases like, "You're not paying attention!" or "Try harder!" No matter how hard you try to get the person to see it, she literally doesn't remember having repeated herself and can't prevent it from happening again.

- **Watch your body language**. When you respond with sighing or eye-rolling, the person "reads" this emotional tone, which can make her feel anxious. The anxiety snowballs into more repetition.

If the loop persists...

- **Try to identify the underlying emotion**—anxiety? boredom? fear?—so you can address your comments accordingly. For example, if she sounds anxious as she's repeating something, you'll want to be extra soothing. If she just seems bored, that's a clue to engage in a fresh activity if you can.

- **Use "bridge phrases" to turn the conversation in a fresh direction**: "Yes, that's a funny story about Rover. *That reminds me of the time we saw the seals at the zoo.*" Or, "*Yes, you fed the animals. Now why don't we pick a TV program?*" Other bridge phrases: *What I'd really like to know is... I've also heard that... Yes, and did you also...* Some people respond well to being diverted to thoughts of an earlier time of life, such as childhood.

- **See if you can identify a trigger that can be removed**. Sometimes a particular dog dish, magazine cover, knick-knack, TV program, or other item trips a thought that gets repeated every time your loved one gazes at it. Moving or getting rid of the prompt might stop the repetition—or, at least, that particular story or question. Rhonda moved the pets' feeding station out of her mother's line of vision, which finally cut down on the questions. My Dad used to read remarkable headlines aloud from the paper. Actually, it was the same headline, over and over. We learned to quickly swap sections whenever he'd get up to replenish his coffee, so we could hear about a different story, for a change.

- **Tell a white lie if you think the answer will soothe**: "Yes, I just fed the animals and they're sleeping happily." Or, to someone who asks, "Where is my mother?" over and over (a not-uncommon expression of anxiety), you might sidestep the truth with a reassuring thought: "She's out right now but gives you this hug. She sure loves you, doesn't she?"

- **Try writing down the answer on a piece of paper**: "We leave for your doctor's appointment at 2 p.m." The next time you're asked, point to the paper. Just having it in hand to look at sometimes curbs further questions.

- **Find an activity that will occupy the person's hands and mind**. This can lessen an underlying emotion causing the repetition (such as boredom or anxiety). Examples: Folding towels, matching socks, polishing silver, organizing a toolbox.

- **Try moving to a different room or starting a new activity**. Distraction can sometimes break the cycle.

- **Consider investing in a digital clock or watch that shows the numbers, along with the date**. If the person with dementia keeps asking the time, she may be finding it challenging to read a clock face.

To help you cope...

- **Try silently counting to 10 before you answer to help calm yourself a notch**. It's natural to be stressed when you're trapped in a conversational loop. Bite your lip. Do deep breathing—anything to distract yourself from reacting to the mounting frustration.

- **Multi-task**. Keeping yourself busy with a project while you talk can make the one-sided nature of the conversation slightly less frustrating.

- **It can sometimes help to leave the room for a few minutes** if you feel like you'll explode. Your absence can be another form of distraction.

o o o

Forgets Recent Visits

When my grandmother could still talk on the phone, early in her Alzheimer's, our conversations would always end the same way: "So when are you coming to see me?"

It didn't matter if I had just been there the day before or an hour before. "When are you coming to see me?" she'd ask in a tone both bright and plaintive.

At least I had it better than some friends, whose parents or grandparents would grow angry: "You never visit me anymore!" Or (to someone who was just there in the morning and went home for lunch): "What took you so long to get here again! You act like you've forgotten all about me!" These are heartbreaking words for a family member who makes a daily visit to a loved one. —P.S.S.

WHY it happens:

Because short-term memory is shot, the encounter doesn't stick in the brain. Repetitive events also tend to run together, so one visit can seem indistinguishable from the next and is less well remembered.

It's helpful to know that, even when your recent presence has been forgotten, the mood boost of having seen you can be huge and outlast your visit by as much as a day or two. Your loved one may not know why she feels happy (from seeing you) but she is.

TRY this:

- **Instead of hearing the comment as an accusation, hear it as an expression of love**. Your relative misses you and looks forward to your time together, whether you've been away for five months or five minutes.

- **Gloss over the complaint**: "Well, I'm here now! Let me tell you about my crazy morning." Or warmly reassure, "I'll visit as often as I can."

- **If you're at a distance, send a calendar** with the date of your next visit as a reminder. It's not a surefire fix, but it's worth a try.

- **Take pictures at each visit, with the date**. When the person complains he or she hasn't seen you lately, you can direct to a photo album to show that you have, which may feel reassuring in the moment. Later, simply looking at pictures of you might be comforting.

- **Vary the events at your visit**. Try bringing balloons one time and a musical instrument the next. This strategy is no guarantee your outings will be better remembered, but each might stand out with more clarity.

- **Whatever you do, avoid arguing**. The person can't follow a logical argument, and your defensiveness will only cause frustration that darkens the mood. The only relevant point is that you're there in that moment, and that moment should be a pleasant experience.

To help you cope:

- **Try to downshift your expectations**. It's not a contest of who's remembered the best. It's all about what happens in the moment.

o o o

Forgets to Take Medication (or Takes It Improperly)

One month Kara noticed that her husband ran out of some of his pills early. In addition to Aricept and Namenda, he takes a beta blocker for high blood pressure, a diuretic, an antidepressant, and several vitamins. She chalked it up to the pharmacy not giving her enough, until her pharmacist, when refilling, assured her that wasn't the case.

The very next day, while vacuuming, she found a couple of pills under a counter near the chair where they usually took their medications in the morning, at breakfast. Maybe he was just dropping them, accidentally or on purpose, she reasoned.

That same week, her daughter Kate brought her two preschoolers over to visit. Kara was enjoying a break in the sunroom when Kate burst in. "Mom! I left the kitchen just for a minute while Dad and the kids were having breakfast together, and when I came back in, he was trying to give them his pills because they thought it was candy!" He was holding his pillbox, trying to open it, when she had walked into the room. Unsure if the kids had swallowed any (they said no and she thought not), she called Poison Control and was told what to watch for. Kara realized he wasn't viewing his medications as drugs any more.

"They wanted some!" he said, when confronted. "It's good to share!"

WHY it happens:

Pill-taking is both a rote task—maybe you take a vitamin every morning after brushing your teeth, without thinking about it—and a complex one. Older adults often have more than one chronic illness, involving multiple drugs that must be taken at a particular time of day, at certain intervals, with or without food, and so on. It's a lot to keep track of.

It's common to forget pills altogether, skip doses, or forget that you've already taken a medicine, and take it twice. Some pill-takers don't notice when a pill falls from the mouth. Or they don't like the taste or size of a pill and spit it out when no one's looking. As their sense of time changes, it can also be harder for them to keep track.

On top of this, people with Alzheimer's sometimes forget how certain objects are used. As in the example of Kara's husband, pills can be mistaken for candy or as a treat or food to be shared with others.

Running out of pills early is a red flag, because it indicates that too many have been taken or lost.

Medication mistakes are a classic early symptom of dementia that can continue and worsen. It's a sign the person can no longer manage this task independently and all aspects of handling medications must be constantly managed and monitored. It would be nice if there were an easy solution. Unfortunately, medication management tends to rest squarely on a family member's shoulders.

TRY this:

- **Make pill-taking part of the daily routine** by linking it with another habit, such as drinking orange juice at breakfast or brushing teeth.

- **Keep a daily log**. Check off when medications are taken, so there's a visual record.

- **Record when a prescription should be filled** (or set up automatic refills). Both measures can help track safe dosing.

- **Bring the pills to the person, rather than counting on him to manage the task**. Watch to make sure they're all swallowed.

- **Consider telephone reminders for mild-stage impairment**. To find a reminder service, enter telephone medication reminder in a search engine. Over time, though, this isn't a reliable way to monitor. You'll need a visual check, actually seeing the person swallow the pill.

For safer dispensing:

- **Switch to a day-of-the-week pillbox if you don't already use one**. There are also versions for a.m./p.m. Some versions lock or have self-timers or alarms, which can help someone early in the disease who's living independently.

- **Look into high-tech dispensers**. This landscape is changing fast, and there are many options. Some send a text or email reminder; others tie into companies, so that if a pillbox isn't opened by a certain time, a call is triggered. It's really important to realize, however, that these methods only work in the earliest stages, and then only for some people. New gadgets are difficult for people with cognitive impairment to master. Often the dispensers' real value is when a message or alert is sent as a reminder to you, the caregiver.

- **Get help getting started**. Pill dispensers only work well if they're properly filled in the first place. A 2011 Northwestern University study found that 60 percent of paid caregivers made errors when sorting meds into pillboxes. Ask the pharmacist to do it for you when prescriptions are filled. Some will do this routinely. Others will do it once or twice to show you how. It can be confounding to figure out what "three times a day" or "every eight hours" looks like in the compartments of a pill organizer. After you get help the first time, draw yourself a "map" of the pills' look and name and where each goes.

- **Fill dispensers at a quiet time when you're feeling alert**. It's not a multitasking kind of job.

Tip: **"Our pharmacist dispensed the pills in blister packs, so you could see if one was taken or not. We'd write the date on the pack above each pill on the pack." —S. K.**

More safety tips:

- **Make sure you understand what each drug is used for and the proper dosing schedule**. You should also know possible side effects to watch for (especially for a new medication).

- **Keep a master list of medications in two places**: on your refrigerator or other central location and in your wallet, so you have it handy at doctor visits. In the event of a hospitalization or specialist appointment, you might be the only person with the complete drug picture.

- **Lock up or store out of reach all extra medications**, as well as other household members' prescriptions, so nothing gets mixed up or taken out of turn. "Out of sight, out of mind" is a good rule of thumb to avoid tempting the person into self-medicating.

- **Ask for a medication review**. Bring all prescription drugs, supplements, and over-the-counter medications used regularly (such as OTC drugs for pain or constipation), in their original containers, to the next primary-care checkup. Ask the doctor to assess whether each is still needed. The fewer meds taken, the fewer to be remembered—and the fewer mistakes or side effects you're likely to encounter. It often makes sense to phase out certain preventative medications as someone ages; Alzheimer's drugs may also prove no longer beneficial as time goes on.

- **For someone who tends to balk at taking pills, offer an incentive**, such as ice cream afterward. Pick a time of day when he or she is most agreeable or well rested, if possible.

- **Check to make sure no pills are too big to be comfortably swallowed**. If so, check with the doctor and/or pharmacist about more manageable alternatives. Some medications can be dispensed in liquid form and then mixed with other foods.

o o o

Forgets to Turn Off Stove

The smell of gas hit Jason as soon as he opened the door to his grandparents' house. His first thought was that there was a leak, and he was about to call the gas company. Once in the kitchen, though, he saw the stove burner on, blue-orange gas flames flicking into the air, with no pot or other sign of cooking in sight.

He quickly turned the burner off, noticing blackened marks around the knobs from previous burns, and opened some windows.

His grandparents were sitting obliviously in the living room, watching TV.

WHY it happens:

Forgetting to turn off the stove can happen to anyone as a result of inattention and preoccupation. Toss in progressive memory loss, and it's a recipe for kitchen danger.

Some people with mild-stage impairment can manage on their own for a while longer, with some safety checks in place. But the inability to use a stove safely or cook is a red flag for being unable to live independently.

TRY this:

- **Consider unplugging a stove**. Plug it in only when someone capable is using it. If the person with dementia can't see the outlet, he or she may not notice what you've done. Another option is to use the shut-off valve (gas stove) or circuit breaker (electric stove).

- **Have a microwave and electric teakettle for use by the person with dementia**. Prepare meals in advance, and put them in separate containers so a single meal's serving can be heated up. A hot water dispenser can be an easy way to provide hot water for soup, tea, or coffee, but it can also be a burn risk. Older skin is more fragile.

- **If you can afford it, look for a replacement stove that has automatic shut-off after a certain period of time**. Timers and motion sensors that detect activity around the stove help prevent accidents.

- **Remove the knobs**. That way, in some models, the stove can't be turned on.

- **To make sure someone who still lives alone is getting essential nutrition**, look into home delivery of meals, through programs such as Meals on Wheels.

o o o

Gets Lost When Driving

Norm liked to drive, and even though his memory problems were getting worse, he seemed to manage a car just fine. One Saturday, he and his wife, Elaine, were out for their usual drive to the farmer's market on the edge of town.

"Norm! You missed the turn!"

Norm looked unconcerned. "We'll just go another way," he said.

Elaine settled back in her seat. After five or 10 minutes, she realized they weren't traveling anywhere near the farmer's market. "Norm, where are we?"

He didn't answer.

"Are you sure this road goes there?"

"I know a shortcut," he said confidently.

After another few minutes, Elaine realized she had no idea where they were and seemed to be traveling in the wrong direction. "But how do we get to the farmer's market from over here?" she persisted.

"Oh, is that where you want to go?" Norm said. "Is it today?"

Elaine then realized that Norm must have forgotten the way well before the first missed turn and they'd been driving aimlessly all this time.

WHY it happens:

Some people with memory loss do well on familiar routes for a while. But there usually comes a day when they miss a turn or lose track of where they were heading. You can't be sure when that day will come. A report on 207 lost drivers with dementia in the *American Journal of Occupational Therapy* points out how dangerous this can be. Only 116 of the lost drivers were found alive, and about a third of those were injured. In another study of 106 drivers with dementia—mostly men in their 50s to 90s who lived with a caregiver—the majority were on errands close to home when they got lost. One in ten were found in a different state!

Backtracking is a complicated cognitive process. Usually the person tends to keep going, sometimes realizing the error and hoping to see a familiar landmark, sometimes continuing obliviously.

TRY this:

- **If the person with dementia has been gone unaccountably long while out driving, contact local law enforcement immediately**. Don't wait several hours to see if he turns up. Most missing older drivers are located by the police. If your state has a Silver Alert system, it can be lifesaving.

- **If it happens just once, with a safe outcome**, thank your lucky stars and consider it a wake-up call that the person can no longer drive safely. Not only his or her life but also the lives of others who are driving, walking, or bicycling on the streets are at risk. As with wandering, once an incident like this happens, it's likely to happen again. It's time to take steps to keep the person from driving, and come up with viable alternatives.

See also in this chapter: "Wanders Off."

o o o

Forgets Someone Died

On the morning after my mother died, after a very short illness, in a hospital bed placed by home hospice in the living room of the house where I grew up, my four siblings and I sat together in the kitchen, our dumbfounded shock still raw. We heard the stairs creak as Dad came down—dressed in a suit. Grim and businesslike, he was ready to go to the funeral home to make arrangements. He often forgot appointments or what he'd just said, but he remembered this important mission. Despite his advancing dementia, he seemed almost like his old self, or at least a grief-stricken version of his usual sunny self.

The next morning, the scene was repeated. Numb siblings, whispered funeral plans over breakfast, and then Dad's footfalls on the staircase. "Good morning," he said in a bright voice. "Are you ready to go see Mother at the hospital?"

"Go see her?"

"She's doing well and sends her love to all of you."

My sisters and I exchanged uneasy glances. "Dad, Mom died two days ago. Remember?"

He burst into tears, stricken anew. "Why didn't anybody tell me? I didn't get to say goodbye!" —P.S.S.

WHY it happens:

This is an extreme yet typical example. People with dementia may express an interest in talking to someone who died years ago, such as a parent, or two days ago (as my dad did). They may be uncertain about the death of a close family member: "Did my brother Bill die?" Or they may be oblivious—for example, talking about inviting Joan and Ralph over to dinner, when Joan or Ralph (or both) died some time ago.

Psychologists have told me that my father (who was deep in middle-stage dementia at the time) was able to recall, the next morning, that his wife had died because the shock of this seismic event was so great. But as time wore on—in this case, less than 48 hours—the fact of her death grew less distinct and more easily forgotten.

Actually it's hard to say whether Dad continued to remember the day of her death in more than a general way, or if it were too painful to go near. After the funeral, he never mentioned my mother (to whom he was married for 67 years and never left the house without kissing) to us again.

TRY this:

- **Gently orient the person when he brings it up**: "Dad, Mom died two days ago." "I'm sorry, Joan was killed in a car crash in 1988."

- **Expect to hear expressions of grief or crying**. These are normal human responses. There's no harm in this. It's not going to make the Alzheimer's any better or worse. Respond to a fresh rekindling of grief with the same empathy and love as you would for a new grief.

- **Brace yourself for no response**. Some people, reminded of a death, say things like, "Oh." Or, "I sure do miss her" and then leave it at that. Or they may say nothing. Don't misconstrue these responses to mean that they didn't love the person. The response they give may be all they're capable of right now. It's okay.

- **Turn the fact of the death into an opportunity for fond reminiscing**: "Wasn't she the sweetest person ever?" "I'll always miss her piano playing. I remember the time she gave that concert at the school...."

- **Don't make a big deal about insisting the person absorb the reality**. There's no need to drive to a cemetery to "prove" the death, show an obituary, etc. Logic is ineffective. Some people will ask follow-up questions, and others will be accepting and not talk about it further.

- **Consider distraction in some situations**. That might be kindest if, for example, the person with dementia becomes fixated on contacting some long-gone relative or wants to buy things for her and can't seem to process the reality of a death.

- **Ultimately, decide what's best in your particular case**. Some families find it easier to tell a little white lie when the questioning is persistent or the person becomes quite agitated every time the topic comes up. It's possible to gloss over the fact, especially as dementia advances. When one woman kept asking about her long-dead husband, her daughter and son would put her off by saying, "He's running late." Or, "He's still on that trip to China" (where their dad in fact once traveled for business). Such comments would pacify her in the moment, and then she'd forget about it. This is a less-good strategy, of course, if your loved one fixates on this falsehood and waits around all day in disappointment.

Should You Tell Someone With Dementia About a Death?

Families often wonder whether to inform someone with dementia of the death of a loved one in the first place. The rationale people give for not saying anything is usually to avoid causing unnecessary distress. Some caregivers say they avoid sharing sad news because they don't want to be asked about it (and have to talk about it or revisit their own grief) over and over.

Most dementia experts agree, though, that the better approach is to be candid. Everyone has a right to know this information, regardless of mental state.

Yes, he or she may have a strong emotional reaction. That's okay. Seeing a household grieving without being told why is also something the person can pick up on and become distressed by. In a nutshell, it's almost always better to know, even if the information is quickly forgotten.

Geri Hall, a wonderful memory-care expert and nurse who has worked at the University of Iowa and the Banner Alzheimer's Institute in Arizona, offers some good advice:

- Tell the person at a time of day that tends to be best for him. Morning? After a meal?

- Make sure the place is free of distractions. TV and radio off, no crowds around.

- It's okay to show emotion yourself. Take the person's hand in yours.

- Establish the context: "I have some sad news about your brother Jack." Don't make it like a quiz. "Do you remember Jack?" But help make clear who you're talking about.

- Don't be surprised if the person with Alzheimer's reacts by trying to comfort you. It's a long-ingrained response. Some people, depending on their faith, culture, and personal mobility, welcome attending a funeral.

"Think about it," Hall says. "If it were you who had dementia, wouldn't you want to know if your loved one had passed?"

o o o

Distorted Sense of Time

In the house where I grew up, the laundry was located in the basement. When my mom would go down to throw in a load, my dad (now with dementia) would quickly grow upset. He'd walk to the top of the stairs and shout down, "What are you doing down there?"

"Laundry!" she'd reply.

A few minutes would pass. He'd go back to the top of the stairs, and slowly make his way down them.

"What?" she'd say.

"I was looking for you," he'd reply.

"I just told you, I was throwing in some wash!"

Conversely, when my Dad went down to the laundry, maybe taking a load from the washer to the dryer, he could be gone for a full hour. Then it was my mom who'd grow curious and creep to the top of the stairs: "Pat! What are you doing down there?" He could fold towels for ages. —P.S.S.

WHY it happens:

Cognitive changes distort the ability to keep track of time. An hour can seem like five minutes. Five minutes can seem like an hour.

TRY this:

- **Be patient**. Your loved one might ask you repeatedly, "What time is it?" or might grow anxious or clingy if you leave the room or are out of sight for several minutes.

- **Know that it's futile to argue**. Same for saying things like, "But we just got here!" or, "I was only gone for two minutes."

- **Make sure clocks are visible in every room the person frequents**. Digital clocks are usually easier to read. This may temporarily reduce anxiety early in dementia. My dad, for example, checked his watch constantly deep into moderate-stage dementia. It seemed to reassure him. But eventually it will grow harder for your loved one to track passing time.

- **Try setting a timer when you have to leave the room**—to go do laundry in the basement, for example. "I'll be back in ten minutes," you might say, "when the bell rings." When you return, be sure to make your presence known. If you do this often, the person gets used to the idea of the bell as a time cue, and may sit patiently by the ticking timer awaiting your return. An old-fashioned hourglass timer that lasts a few minutes works, too.

- **Try to always be prompt or early**. Don't stay away or out of sight longer than you said you would. Announce your return.

- **Check in periodically in person or by voice when you're both around the house**. It's reassuring and the other person may be less apt to miss you.

- **Keep a large calendar in a central area where you can record appointments**. Review it in the morning (and as needed through the day) to reassure the person that he won't miss any important events.

- **Try to stretch out time with a distraction when you're out in public** and the person insists after just five minutes, "I want to go home." You can say, "Just a few more minutes. We're about to hear some music/look at some pictures/have some coffee." Realize, though, that if he or she grows more agitated, the simplest course may be to try again another day.

- **Structure the day around a solid routine**. The predictable flow of activities—meals, a walk, TV time, nap, and so on—helps mark the passage of the day even when a clock can't be read.

o o o

Doesn't Recognize Familiar People

Toward the end of his life, my father was living in a nursing home for rehabilitation following a small stroke. At every visit, he'd reach for a copy of Woman's Day *magazine, which he kept on his bedside table. For years, I'd been a columnist for the magazine, writing about family.*

He'd hand me the magazine, pointing to my picture on a carefully bookmarked page. "Have you read Paula's new article?"

He knew I was familiar. He referred to my name. He knew, I'm pretty sure, that I was family. But which family, exactly, had grown muddled. He often introduced me to the nursing staff (who knew me) by saying, "Have you met my sister?" or "This is my sister, Betty." But then he'd ask after my children, his grandchildren, sometimes by name.

There's nothing quite like the astonishment that grabs you the first time this person you've known your entire life can't quite place you. I felt an odd mix of understanding and disbelief.

Dad always seemed to know I was a person who loved him, and— for both of us—that had to be enough. —P.S.S.

WHY it happens:

The inability to recognize friends and family—even a spouse or adult child—is a byproduct of declining memory.

Often it's a matter of "last to know, first to go." Those who entered the person's life later, including grandchildren, sons- or daughters-in-law, some colleagues, tend to be forgotten before siblings, for example. Names tend to slip first. (My dad often asked, "How's the family?" to cover for the fact that he wasn't sure which of us had children and who they were.) Your loved one may know that a certain face is familiar without being able to state the exact relationship.

Familiar people get confused with others, too. It's not unusual for someone with Alzheimer's to mistake his adult daughter for his wife, for example—even to the point of making advances.

It's important to understand what are NOT reasons for this confusion: You're not forgotten because you weren't around enough, weren't emotionally close enough, or aren't loving or giving enough now. Being forgotten or confused for another isn't a reflection on you or the quality of your relationship, now or in the past.

TRY this:

- **At first, gently offer the correct name or relationship, if you like**: "Actually I'm Paula, his daughter," I'd say to the staff after being mis-introduced. "You've always said I look like Betty, haven't you, Dad?" Or I'd call him "Dad" a lot to re-orient him. Just try to do it in a way that preserves the person's dignity.

- **Ultimately, you have to let it pass**. If he keeps forgetting or truly seems to have no idea who you are, let it go. ("Yup, I've read all her articles," I'd say of the magazine columnist Paula, a.k.a. me.) It doesn't really matter.

- **Pre-empt trouble by offering a prompt when you see him**: "Hi, Dad, it's Paula, your favorite middle daughter!" "Look who's come to see you, your bowling buddy Norm!"

- **Forewarn friends or those who haven't seen the person in a while**. Better they're prepared.

- **Avoid turning it into a test**. My dad (before his own dementia was obvious) used to quiz his mother-in-law, who had Alzheimer's and knew no one by the end: "Do you know me? How about her—do you know who this is?" That puts unnecessary stress on the person with memory loss. (With little knowledge about dementia, he seemed truly befuddled that she could forget everyone.)

- **If the person behaves inappropriately—for example, a father making a pass at a daughter—avoid blowing it out of proportion**. Remember the "why." Instead, stay calm and distract the person, then redirect the behavior to something else. "I have an idea, let's go get some chocolate." "I'm tired; how about a walk in the fresh air?"

To help you cope:

- **Realize that your presence is felt and matters!** People sometimes think, "Why should I bother visiting? He doesn't even know me." But even after names and relations are lost to the person, close relationships still register as beloved, familiar figures. Your presence is cheering, comforting, and de-stressing. A rose still smells sweet, even if you don't know what that pretty pink fragrant thing that cheers you up is called.

o o o

CONFUSING COMMUNICATION

Here's an illustration of just how hard it can be to adjust your ways of talking to someone in a world re-colored by dementia. Both my husband and I had experience with relatives' dementia and we'd both worked in the eldercare field. Yet when my father-in-law came to live with us at age 93, we were slow to attribute his occasional delusions and other behavior changes to what we later learned was frontotemporal dementia—largely because his symptoms didn't match what we'd seen before in other family members—and we were slower still to respond effectively. A typical exchange:

"So, are you calling me a cab?"

"A cab?" (He hadn't ridden in a taxi for over 10 years.) "Why? Where do you need to go?"

"To see MY WIFE!"

"But Dad, Mom died two years ago."

"I got married again four weeks ago!"

"But you haven't left the house in four weeks. How could we have missed that?"

"Her son the minister married us!"

"Really? Where is she now?"

"At the motel! I need to go there!"

"Which motel is it?"

"Oh....Camcorder! Camcorder Inn or something."

"That can't be it. Let's eat dinner while we try to figure it out."

"Oh, I can't eat. I'm too upset. I couldn't keep anything down!"

What Helps in General

Here are some basics that can pave the way to smoother, happier communication for all:

To lessen frustration all around, avoid correcting, reasoning, and arguing:

- **Be ready for even ordinary conversations to go off the rails quickly**, and not always for reasons you can control. Patience, that scarce resource for those living with dementia, can pull you back from the edge if you can muster it. Remember: Though it sounds like your familiar family member's or friend's voice, it's dementia doing the talking.

- **Instead of addressing their faulty facts, play back the emotions you're sensing**. This helps the person with dementia feel understood. "You sound anxious to get there." "You look sad."

- **To avoid going down a rabbit hole of confused logic, respond with generalities**. Great ones: "Really?" "I didn't know that." "Maybe." "Well, let's see what happens." "I'll let you know." "Tell me more about that."

- **Agree...with a postponement**. "Okay, I'll do it this afternoon." "Sure, after I finish this." "You're right. Let's plan it later." Sometimes the person simply wants to be heard in the moment, and thus pacified, will promptly forget a request or brewing argument.

- **Keep in mind that speaking tone usually matches the words being said**. So when you're correcting, you sound irritated—and the person picks up on that and gets more agitated.

To aid the brain's slowing processor, slow down and simplify:

- **When initiating a conversation, first make a connection**. Approach someone with mid-stage Alzheimer's from the front, so you're less likely to surprise. Avoid starting a conversation by calling from across the room. Get into the person's line of vision. Crouch to a seated person's level, for example. Make eye contact. Use body language (a gentle touch on the forearm or back) to avoid startling.

- **Slow your rate of speech a little bit to give more time for your words to sink in**. You don't have to exaggerate the slowdown. Just don't rush.

- **Break ideas into one thought at a time**. Break directions into small, discrete steps. Break sentences into fewer words. One thing at a time. Less is more.

- **Refrain from rushing to fill silences**. Give the person a chance to come up with a word or thought, as much as is feasible.

- **If you have to repeat yourself, try pausing and then use the exact same words**. ("Would you like lunch? ... Would you like lunch?") That helps the person process. It's harder to follow the same question asked three slightly different ways in rapid-fire order. ("Would you like lunch?" "Do you want to eat now?" "Hey, are you hungry yet or do you want to eat later?")

- **Reduce background noise when you're trying to talk**. The radio or TV can be distracting or just hard to hear over.

To gently help orient the person, use conversational crutches:

- **Weave in references to people you introduce, talk about, or point out in photos:** "Look, here's your son Jack." "Your friend Alice from the club says...."

- **Use consistent labels for things every time you mention them:** "the blue pill box," "your next-door neighbor Bob," "your favorite sweet-smelling tea." Avoid vague words like *this* and *over there*.

- **Early in the disease, try written guides that underscore your spoken words**. Put labels on shelves and cupboards: hand towels, bath towels, sheets. Some people find very simple lists of instructions helpful, or like to keep notepads handy to jot down their thoughts.

- **Skip phrasings that feel like a test or that put the person on the spot**. Avoid asking, "Do you know me today, Dad?" "You remember Alice, don't you?" "Who's this?"

To boost mood and cooperation, offer a measure of control:

- **Ask. Don't tell**. Instead of, "Let me do that," try, "Can I help you with that?" or "Hmm, may I try?"

- **Offer choices**. Everybody likes to exert his or her opinions. It feels good! Make it a choice between two things, though:

"Do you want the red or blue shirt?" Tip: If you have a preference, offer the choice you prefer last, as it will most likely be the one accepted. Simplest are yes/no questions: "Do you want to wear your blue shirt today?" Keep in mind, though, that eventually any kind of choosing may prove too stressful.

- **Rely on a roster of phrases to smooth over rough patches**: "Everything has been taken care of." "I'm sorry you're upset." "I know it's hard." "You're in good hands with me!

- **Even if it gets old for you, return to topics that the person has shown he or she relates to and enjoys**. Maybe it's the weather, the birds at the feeder, or sports. As deterioration goes on, current events and pop culture may become frustrating to follow because they demand more short-term memory, abstract reasoning, and concentration.

To better match the person's reality, sidestep the truth as needed:

- **"Give" in fantasy what you can't in reality**: "Oh I wish we could go to your momma's house right this minute. Let's plan what we'd do there." Try sparking a conversation that soothes over the present moment; the plans will be quickly forgotten but the sense of pleasure can persist. "Oh I wish I could give you 20 ice cream cones! Wouldn't that be yum; what are your favorite flavors?"

- **Leave out information that might be contentious**. Bob DeMarco of Alzheimer's Reading Room tells how he learned not to tell his mother it was time for a bath. Instead he'd offer her an outstretched hand and say, "Let's go." "Where?" she'd ask. "To have fun," he'd say. That put her in a pleasant mood, from which he'd walk her step by step through the process and promise ice cream afterwards. (That part was no fib.)

- **Blame circumstances, whether they're true or not**. When Don, my father-in-law, insisted on visiting his imagined wife in the hospital one evening, my husband told him he called the hospital and was told visiting hours had just ended. Don fumed at the "stupid hospital" for a few minutes, but let it go.

To make everything go better, don't forget nonverbal communication!

- **Use your body language to underscore your message**. Think about the difference a smile or calm expression makes to you, compared to a furrowed brow, narrowed eyes, clenched fists, hunched shoulders, and other signs of frustration or anger.

- **Use gestures**. Some people are quicker to understand when you pantomime a little. For example, point to the kitchen when you say, "Lunch is ready." Pretend to drink from an imaginary cup while you ask, "Are you thirsty?"

- **"Listen" to the body language of the person with dementia, too**. Their general mood (contentment, anxious, pained) may not match the words they're using.

- **Feed the sense of touch**. Older adults, especially widowed ones, are often deprived of human touch. A hand on a shoulder or elbow, holding hands, or rubbing a shoulder while you converse can be calming and make your message better received.

- **Remember this**: Sometimes a hug is the best way to say anything.

o o o

Repetition

See Memory Problems section: "Repeats Same Questions or Comments Within Minutes (or Less)"

Can't Find the Right Words

Zelda stood in front of her daughter with her hands on her hips. "Where's my, my—my read."

"Read?" her daughter, Zoe, asked, blankly.

"Box! Read box. You know, my read box! I just had it."

"Breadbox?"

Zelda shook her head. "Of course not, silly! You know what I mean!"

"Mom, I don't. Read box? You mean like a Kindle? You don't have one, Mom. Would you like to have a tablet to read books?"

Zelda finally spotted her paperback on the kitchen table. "Oh, here it is."

WHY it happens:

Trouble finding the right word is a common early sign of Alzheimer's, since both memory and parts of the brain used for speech and language are affected. This is called aphasia. (Not everyone with Alzheimer's has it.) Primary progressive aphasia (PPA) is a form of frontotemporal dementia. Aphasia is also common with stroke victims and those who also have vascular dementia (caused by small strokes or blood vessel disease).

Aphasia gets progressively worse, although the rate of decline is different for each person. It affects not only word choice but also the ability to speak clearly, understand others, read, and write. Some people have trouble in one of these areas but not others. At first, for example, someone may have trouble finding words, but reasoning and visual perception involved with reading and writing are still intact. Spelling and math problems (such as writing numerals or adding them) are related effects.

What you might hear:

- Hesitancy and long pauses in the middle of a sentence as the person searches for the word

- A generic term substituted for any word, such as *thingamabob, stuff, thingy, that-there* (*white stuff* for salt, *black stuff* for pepper)

- Substitution of a word or phrase that's somehow related (so *read box* for book, *writing stick* for pencil, *mouth cleaner* for toothbrush)

- Substitution of a similar-sounding word or made-up word (*kappy* for kitty, *launch* for lunch, *sweer* for shower)

- Getting stuck on a word and repeating it over and over

- Stringing together lots of nonsense words or gibberish

- Words whispered or spoken so softly that you can barely hear them, much less make them out

- You might also notice that someone who has trouble speaking may still be able to understand what's said to her.

TRY this:

- **Don't get caught up in trying to "teach" the correct word or make a big deal about mistakes**. Sometimes the goofs are pretty funny, but to avoid embarrassment, laugh only if self-deprecating humor or lightness is part of the person's personality and your relationship.

- **Early on, give the speaker some space to come up with the right word**. If you rush in to supply it, you add to frustration. If she's really foundering, wait a few seconds, then go ahead and supply what you think she means. "Oh, your book? It's on your chair." Or say, "Your book? Am I on the right track?"

- **Try rolling with it**. Educator Anne Basting, who uses a lot of verbal play in her work, told me a great story of a man whose wife grew frustrated when she couldn't recall the word for ketchup. He said, "Well, what do you want to call it? Let's make up a word together." And so they called it *red sauce*. That kind of thinking is freeing to the person with dementia: Instead of just one "right" answer and 1,000 wrong ones, you've opened things up to where there are 1,000 different right answers.

- **Make it your problem**. Social worker and Alzheimer's expert Joyce Simard often blames herself when asking someone to repeat. "I'm sorry, my hearing isn't so good. What did you say?"

- **Listen beyond just the words**. Pay attention to gesturing and body language, as well as the context of the rest of the sentence, to discern meaning.

Tip: "Mom took to carrying around a notebook in which she'd write down questions or comments for us. She had a lot of trouble talking, but early on, she could still write, and it eased her frustration." —J.R.

- **Speak slowly, and focus on getting just one idea across at a time**. ("Let's eat lunch," not "After lunch we'll go to the store for your art supplies.")

- **Try introducing creative arts such as music or painting**. Some research shows that many people whose language capacity shrinks enjoy creative outlets they never had (or even showed an interest in) before. Singing, making things, or playing an instrument can become means of self-expression. It makes sense, given how the arts rely on metaphor.

- **Consider seeing a speech pathologist or occupational therapist** who has experience working with dementia patients. Especially early in the disease, or after a stroke, they can often help find new ways to communicate.

- **Create "I have aphasia cards" to discreetly hand out in public**. The National Stroke Association recommends carrying cards that say something like, "My mother has aphasia, which means she can't speak well or understand speech well. Please speak clearly and slowly. Thanks for your patience."

To help you cope:

- **Know that your patience may be sorely tested because these speech changes can be maddening, confusing, and even scary**. But getting upset will only make your companion upset. Realize that this is a frustrating and frightening development for him or her. Reach out with added hugs, physical contact, and supportiveness to help her feel more loved and connected despite the wedge of a language barrier.

o o o

Talks to Himself or Herself

"Thank you, General of the Army. Now that I'm a major general, I'm going to promote my good wife to brigadier general...Well you have the authority, General...ha ha ha...All right you can kiss the brigadier general...good, good...well your wife could be promoted too...ha ha ha...

"You know what I haven't had in a long time? Ham and eggs. Why my butcher friend is waving to me. I bet he has something in mind. He says this Monday we're having a big sale on all those meats...Okay, I'm glad you told me that...we'll make 15 to 18 percent on them...I understand. We'll do our part and fill up the old freezer again. Turkeys, too?...Oh, those are for next season, he says.

"I'm sorry to say, I cannot perform...all the other fellas have to step in for me. I'm sorry. I. Am. Ill. Oh, I wanna lie down and I'm gonna lie down, so help me ....Now, what the heck time of day is it? If they fire me, they fire me. I want to do my level best. But I'm ashamed to say, I cannot perform...

"She said, Honestly, tell me now, did you ever touch anyone in the cookery?...I never touched a gal in the cookery!...Okay, I was wrong...You sure as hell were. I'll try to keep my so-called indiscretions to myself...."

All these are verbatim comments by my father-in-law. He'd talk to himself for hours while sitting in the backyard, in his room—or, later, right in front of us. (I couldn't help writing them down as they became more incredible.) Sometimes they seemed rooted in reality—talk about what he liked to eat or stories from his childhood. Just as often, though—and sometimes veering from reality to delusion without missing a beat—he'd narrate back-and-forth conversations with another person, supplying both voices. At times he talked the part of a college baseball recruit, a hair-salon owner, a construction contractor, a general, a four-time married man—nothing that had happened in his real life, by any stretch.

Most astonishing was the time he "narrated" the (again completely made-up) rape trial of a granddaughter, playing by turns the voices of the judge, the lawyers, and all the witnesses! He even played someone who sounded like me, with true-life details sprinkled in: "Your Honor, this is my second marriage. I have three daughters and a son from my first marriage. Jim, my current husband, is by far the best man I've ever known. He is not lying when he told you...."

Even more amazing: He'd never been a talker, actor, raconteur, or storyteller of any kind earlier in life! —P.S.S.

WHY it happens:

Some people have always talked to themselves, keeping it in their heads or at a low mutter. For others this is a new habit. Either way, as self-control (inhibition) decreases, the filter that kept us from talking aloud disappears, and verbalizations come out at anytime, anywhere, any volume. When it's constant, this behavior is known as verbal agitation.

Talking to yourself can have a purpose for anyone. It can be a way to help remember things, to walk yourself through steps, or to reassure yourself. It can be purely entertaining (as in the examples above), especially if the person lacks for companions. It can be a way to work through different emotions or make sense of random thoughts (probably also the case for my father-in-law). Not that it's always easy to listen to!

Early self-talking can seem to have purpose and logic. But as time goes on, the talk may sound increasingly disjointed or nonsensical.

TRY this:

- **Tune out what you can**. Once this kind of self-talk is incessant, don't feel you need to respond to it. Turning a deaf ear is okay. Wear headphones when you need to concentrate.

- **Listen for messages within the words**. The person may not be talking to you but may nevertheless be communicating about pain or another state. Listen to the tone. Is it jovial? Sad? Worried? Look for patterns. Some people use self-talk more when they're anxious, for example, or do it more in the evening. (See later in this chapter: "Sundowning.")

- **Consider adding social outlets**. If you're tapped out on the talking, hiring an elder companion (or finding a volunteer) to sit and listen to stories can help meet an unmet social need.

- **Redirect with something you know the person likes**: watching a ball game, eating ice cream, listening to music. Or offer the person something to eat: gum (if safe) or a lollypop that can occupy the mouth for long periods.

To help you cope:

- **Give your ingrained instinct for politeness a break**. It can feel unkind, even unnatural, to ignore someone speaking. When your sanity is at stake, remind yourself this isn't really about having a dialogue.

- **Try developing a signal if the talk veers into the unacceptable**. My father-in-law's tales sometimes turned X-rated, and our house was often full of teenagers. Sometimes a sharp rap on his door would disrupt him, although this lost effectiveness as time went on. We finally put a radio nearby to replace the drone with music.

o o o

Uses Nonsense Words, Gibberish

"Hey diddlie diddle, do do do do," Lucille croons to herself as she rocks in her usual armchair. "Do do majig."

"How are you today, Mama?" asks her husband, Bill. They've been married for 63 years.

"Diddlie diddle. I want my majiggy jig," Lucille responds.

Bill has no idea what she's saying. "Yes, love, I'm going to make our lunch right now with your favorite brownies for dessert," he says. He kisses the top of her head as he passes by.

WHY it happens:

Language that doesn't make sense is an extreme kind of aphasia—or loss of language—caused by dementia. This particular loss tends to show up in later stages. The person loses the ability to find the right words and express them.

Speech may be a mix of nonsense words and a few that make sense, garbled-sounding real speech, or purely nonsensical.

This speech pattern can also become an almost involuntary self-soothing habit. She calms herself down through this kind of talk. Some people only use nonsense speech when tired and trying to sleep.

TRY this:

- **Avoid urging the speaker to try to be clearer**. She literally can't try any harder.

- **Study the body language to help you figure out a meaning**. Agitated rocking? Humming and smiling? Wandering around looking for something?

- **See if you can connect a mood to the speech**, either through the tone used or the circumstances. Someone who can't find something or doesn't want to go somewhere might mutter angrily, for example.

- **Respond differently as needed**. Show added love and reassurance if the gibberish seems to increase when your loved one is upset, lonely, or bored.

To help you cope:

- **Find conversational outlets**. Listening to gibberish can be stressful and make the person seem remote, so it can really help to have others in your life you can truly talk to.

- **Don't worry too much about trying to interpret exactly what she's trying to say**. Like Bill in the example above, you may need to just go with the flow. Stick to a routine and try to anticipate needs that can't be communicated (time to be hungry for lunch?).

o o o

Asks, "What Should I Be Doing?"

An aide wheels my mother-in-law into the sunny dining room where she lives with her husband and my sister-in-law and her family. It's a holiday, and everyone's just sitting around, relaxed.

"How are you today?" someone asks.

"I'm fine," she assures. "What should I be doing?"

"You don't need to do anything, Mom," her daughter tells her. "Paula and Jim are here visiting, and we're going to have lunch soon."

"Oh, okay." Then, a few minutes later she asks her husband: "What should I be doing? Is there something I should be doing?" —P.S.S.

WHY it happens:

Humans have an inborn need to be busy, to contribute. This feeling is especially strong among those who have been active all their lives, working and/or looking after others. At the same time, loving, well-meaning family caregivers tend to want to make life easy for the person with Alzheimer's. We do as much as we can for them. Sometimes, that's too much.

Without a task or responsibility to manage, a child to raise, a job to tend, your loved one may have little or nothing to do. Yet she still feels a lingering sensation that she should be doing something. Feelings tend to live longer and stronger than memories. It's like that haunting sense you get when you walk into a room intending to do something, but once you're there, you can't put your finger on what it was.

Confusion, boredom, and anxiety can bring these feelings to the fore. When the person is frail and physically unable to do much, the problem is intensified.

TRY this:

- **Look for ways to involve the person in meaningful activities rather than doing every little thing for him or her**. The smallest acts, even things you'll wind up having to re-do later, can fill the bill. The definition of "meaningful" will change over time as mental and physical abilities change. It doesn't have to be much to provide the satisfying feelings of contributing.

- **Consider reserving one or two particular tasks that match his or her ability**. Taking ownership of a chore can underscore a sense of purpose. Maybe your mom always sets the table or folds the laundry. Maybe your dad brings in the mail (if wandering isn't a potential issue).

- **Remind yourself to ask for help**. We all love to be sought after and included. Ask her help when tying a ribbon on a package or stirring a soup. Or simply solicit her opinion on whether the soup needs salt or which color of ribbon looks best on the gift you're wrapping.

- **Focus on what the person can do now, not what she once did**. Maybe your mom can no longer bake her special oatmeal cookies. But perhaps she can "coach" you in the steps (even though she may not remember them and you'll be the one guiding her along). Or you can give her slice-and-bake dough to form on cookie sheets, a familiar act.

- **Don't worry about programming every minute of the day**. Just try to weave some interesting activities into the daily routine. This stamps out boredom and brings purpose to the day.

o o o

Curses (But Didn't Used to) or Says Other Mean, Hurtful, or Inappropriate Things

"You cheap SOB!" Elizabeth raged at Frank, her husband of 49 years. "Why don't you buy me some new clothes, you f---ing bastard!" For most of her life, the elegant and well-bred Elizabeth was soft-spoken and unfailingly polite. Frank always admired how she knew just the right thing to say in any circumstance.

"The first time she cursed, she said 'dammit' under her breath when she was having trouble getting out of the car," Frank says. "That alone was kind of shocking. But I figured it was because she was upset by her Alzheimer's diagnosis." Then she began hurling swear words behind his back, often when she didn't want to do something he asked her to do, like take a bath, eat dinner, or go to bed. As the years went on the sailor-talk became louder and more frequent. Mostly, these outbursts have been targeted at poor Frank.

"She has all the clothes she could want, I'm gentle, I don't deny her anything," he says with sadness. "She makes up a lot of indignities and hurls the most horrible words at me—words I never knew she'd even heard!"

WHY it happens:

Swearing is rarely intentional in someone who has dementia, especially when it's a new behavior for the person. It's surprisingly common, though, for mild-mannered people to begin using salty phrases they never before uttered.

A healthy person might think something crude when angry but not voice it. We're taught not to do so as children, and these messages are reinforced by the norms of polite society. As adults, we then automatically self-censor things we know not to be appropriate (at least, as best we can, though not always in bad traffic!). In dementia, however, there's damage to the part of the brain's processing centers involved in self-control. The person becomes less able to regulate certain behaviors, including language.

Swearing is often triggered by anger, frustration, or fear. Interestingly, there's research to show that even in healthy people, occasional cursing is a way to cut the sensation of pain.

The loss of self-control in dementia (called disinhibition) can also cause someone to use uncharacteristically crude words, belch or pass gas loudly, holler nonsense, wail, make random animal sounds, or say rude comments. (One caregiver reports his wife would make a low "moo" sound whenever she saw an obese person in public.)

TRY this:

- **At first, draw a line:** "Please don't talk to me like that, Jane." "That's not a very nice word." Then distract to another activity or conversation. But if the chiding doesn't work and the cursing continues, simply ignore it.

- **Avoid dramatic shushing or shaming**. Try not to act shocked or startled. It can make someone with dementia feel bad or even fuel more of the behavior, without solving the problem. Better: React with calm indifference.

- **Look for an underlying trigger**: Is your loved one feeling stressed? Bored? Upset about something? Is it too noisy, for example, or are children speaking faster than the person with dementia can understand? Addressing the cause of the emotion can often end a bout of potty mouth.

- **One way to find a trigger is to look for patterns**. Does the meanness tend to come out at certain times, such as during bathing? Maybe there's something about the experience that's upsetting, like your loved one is getting chilled without your realizing it. Bob DeMarco, the founder of Alzheimer's Reading Room, noticed his mother would hurl hurtful language his way whenever he'd been talking on the phone. He eventually figured out that she believed he was talking to someone about putting her in a "home," one of her fears. Long detailed explanations that this wasn't true were of no use. What worked: Being extra loving and reassuring with hugs and words after he hung up, then distracting with a pleasant activity.

- **In public, you can apologetically and discreetly explain that the cursing is an unfortunate behavior caused by her dementia**. Some families have business cards made to discreetly hand to wait staff, store clerks, or others in public settings: "Please excuse my [wife/mother]. She has dementia, which causes her to act in unpredictable ways."

- **If children overhear, give an age-appropriate explanation**. For example, "Grandma has a sickness in her brain that makes her talk funny and say bad words. She never used them before she got sick, and you shouldn't either."

- **Mention a tough case to the doctor**. Certain medications or drug interactions can increase disinhibition in some people.

To help you cope:

- **Let yourself grieve**. This behavior can be distressing to witness and endure.

- **Don't make the common mistake of assuming the epithets are your loved one's "real personality"** or "true feelings about you" coming out. Even if the swearing is directed at you personally, it's usually a response to how she's feeling in the moment about something going on.

- **Know that using vulgar language can be one of those intractable behaviors where the best you can do is to "grin and bear it."** Some caregivers use humor to cut the discomfort: "Oh, Sue, you sound like someone in an R-rated movie!"

o o o

Says, "I Want to Go Home"

As my grandmother's Alzheimer's progressed, she'd sit in a quiet stupor for most of our visits to the nursing home. She'd moved there two years earlier, after breaking a hip at age 97. At some point, on some days, she'd suddenly perk up: "Are we going home? Where's my purse? Have we paid yet?"

She seemed to think we were in a restaurant. And we'd all freeze, unsure what to say. "Gram, this isn't Red Lobster," would only confuse her. So did explaining that this place was her home. (I tried that once and she said, "Like hell.") Usually she'd just get adamant: "Bring me my purse so I can pay. I'm ready to go home now." — P.S.S.

Why it happens:

In the language of Alzheimer's, "going home" usually expresses a desire for security. Home is a warm, fuzzy, happy concept for most of us, a place of refuge and nurturing. Think of the expressions, "home is where the heart is," "hearth and home," "home sweet home." Also, memories held the longest are those of earlier life. These are often happy memories of growing up or of a beloved community.

The person may be feeling some kind of discomfort and longing for the security that "home" represents. Maybe she's confused because she doesn't recognize where she is (whether it's her own longtime residence, a care community, or a temporary stay at a hospital). She may be anxious about something (a visit she senses is coming to an end, an upcoming shower or bed bath). Some people also talk about going home when they're tired.

TRY this:

- **Skip trying to orient the person by saying, "But you are home!" or "This is your home now."** The intellectual capacity to reason is gone. Trying to re-orient will likely lead to more confusion or argument.

- **Hear home as a feeling your loved one needs you to understand**. Too often someone with dementia is told "you are home," but the underlying emotional need goes unaddressed. So the person grows more distressed.

- **Instead, try hearing "I want to go home" as "I'm uneasy" or "I'm scared."** Try meeting the emotional need—fear, uncertainty—with an upbeat little fib that meets the person where she is, while reassuring: "The weather's too cold now, maybe later." "Why don't we listen to some music first?" Some people with dementia believe they're at a hotel, restaurant, cruise ship, or other trip-related setting, and caregivers go along with this idea: "We'll go back home soon, maybe tomorrow."

  "A fib-let is better than a tablet," says caregiver advocate and former spousal caregiver Joanne Koenig Coste, author of Learning to Speak Alzheimer's.

- **Offer reassurance in the form of a hug**. Body language is often effective where words and logic won't work. Satisfy the need to feel secure.

- **Use verbal reinforcement**. At random times, say things like, "I feel so safe and happy living in this nice house." "You're safe with me, kiddo." (Avoid using these responses in direct argument to "I want to go home," though.)

- **Pay attention to care circumstances that might be triggering the discomfort**. Does the person talk about going home at certain times, such as before bedtime? Is there something distressing about her routine at this time (for example, does she dislike showering or have a new care aide who makes her uncomfortable)? This expression isn't necessarily a condemnation of a living situation, but it's worth double-checking for possible problems. Many can be easily fixed and improve quality of life.

- **Don't bend over backward making a reunion visit to a home place**. Remember, someone with dementia rarely means home literally. She may be thinking of a place she lived in a long time ago, such as her birthplace or the house where she raised her family. Or all the happy places she's lived may be co-mingling in her mind to represent a vague, satisfying feeling, not an actual place. While such a trip can be fun (if she's physically capable), you have to brace for the possibility that even a visit to an intact old home won't satisfy the longing that's been expressed. If the place is gone or altered, even if your family member can remember it, she may be even more confused.

- **If the person is insistent about getting in the car or "going now," try this**. Go for a drive (such as around the block or out for ice cream). Pull back up to her current residence and cheerfully announce, "We're home!"

- **Use home as a springboard for distracting conversation**. "You really miss home. Tell me about it." Ask about favorite activities or places "back home" or what she'll do first when she "gets home."

- **Go home with photos**. Look at old pictures from the stage of life your loved one seems to have happy memories about. My father (who seemed to think his new home in my younger brother's house was a cruise ship) could look at a childhood snapshot of his hometown and describe the name of every family in the tiny houses in the background. Don't do this intending to orient: "See, this is your home! This old one was burned down, remember?" Instead, do it as a way to placate: "We can't go home yet, but look at these pictures I found. Let's look at them and plan our trip."

To help you cope...

- **Separate your emotions from what's being said**. Hearing, "I want to go home," can provoke many feelings: worry that a loved one is unhappy in a given setting, guilt at having made an out-of-home placement, disappointment or anger that your loved one sounds unsatisfied by all the sacrifices you're making on her behalf. Those who have taken in an adult parent may fear that it means they haven't done enough to make the parent feel at home. Keep in mind that someone with dementia isn't likely to be making jibes to manipulate you.

o o o

HELP-RELATED ISSUES

Resists Seeing a Doctor

The whispers among M.J.'s family members grew more urgent: What's up with Mom? Have you noticed? M.J., who lived half a mile away, was the first to notice. Her two sisters across the state finally agreed they couldn't ignore the funny behaviors any more—how Mom mixed up two grandchildren's names, the day Mom had her second fender bender in a week, the time she showed up for a family dinner but had the day wrong.

"Mom, you feeling okay?" they'd ask.

"I'm fine. Your poor old ma is just getting older," Adele, their mother, would say.

Then she knocked over her daughter's mailbox while backing down the drive, during a visit in which she'd forgotten the year her husband died, and the cookies she'd made were oddly inedible. All small things? M.J., a nurse, knew otherwise.

The girls sat her down together to insist she get checked out. Adele flatly denied there was a problem. She blamed the car accident on the weather (as she had the previous two incidents) and the cookies on "a bad batch of flour." If ever she acknowledged a misstep at all (she often didn't), there was always an excuse—a headache, a lousy receptionist, bad drivers, and her favorite, "You misheard me."

WHY it happens:

Someone with symptoms might resist seeing a doctor because of:

- *Dread:* She suspects a brain-related illness, but the stigma of Alzheimer's is enough to make her play ostrich and ignore it. (That's likely, since Alzheimer's is the second most feared disease, after cancer.)

- *Procrastination:* She's aware that she's making mistakes and having trouble with thinking skills but hopes the problem will clear up and go away.

- *Denial:* She truly doesn't see it as a problem that merits a doctor's attention—the "just old age" rationale.

- *Dislike of medical care:* She avoids doctors generally.

- *Obliviousness:* Her case is advanced to the point where she fails to recognize a problem.

To all this, add the complexities of how it feels when other people in your life tell you what you *should* do (get to a doctor). When the message comes from adult children, a parent may feel it's "not your business." Even when the message comes from a spouse, there can be a resistance borne in dread, that the person you trust most is confirming your deepest fear. And some prickly personality types perceive any suggestions as nagging.

Most cases of dementia of all kinds actually go undiagnosed, says the U.S. Preventive Services Task Force. Mostly, this is because people don't get screened or evaluated in the first place. Usually aware of a problem at first, they avoid the doctor or don't take symptoms seriously. Family members, too, can get in the way of a health evaluation. A 2012 study by the Alzheimer's Foundation of America found that two-thirds of those who saw behavioral symptoms of Alzheimer's in a loved one felt they were "just a normal part of aging." (They weren't.) Of these, 67 percent said that such thinking delayed getting a diagnosis.

Sometimes doctors miss the signs because the person pulls it together for the duration of the exam. In one small study from 2000, 11 in 14 people found to have mild dementia had no record of it in their medical charts; nor did five in seven of those with moderate dementia or one in five with severe dementia.

With today's improved screenings, doctors can make a probable diagnosis of Alzheimer's with as much as 95 percent certainty.

TRY this:

- **Start by believing in the benefits of early diagnosis.** What's the big deal about putting a name to the problem? Does it matter if you know the exact reason Mom is forgetful or Dad gets lost driving? As with any health matter, it's best to know exactly what you're dealing with. Memory loss, poor judgment, and other symptoms aren't natural byproducts of getting older. Nor do they necessarily mean Alzheimer's. Many conditions mimic Alzheimer's. By having a professional opinion on what's normal or not, you can get reversible problems treated.

   And if it is a form of dementia? Starting lifestyle changes and treatments sooner, including medications, rather than later, can slow impairment. Knowing what you're dealing with gives you a chance to learn about the course of the disease, so you're not always blindsided. An early diagnosis can make the person eligible for, and able to benefit from, clinical trials. You can also find out about community resources. And knowing early gives the affected person a valuable chance to have input on important decisions before it's too late.

It's true that you don't need an official diagnosis or label to help manage daily life with dementia. The issues you deal with will mostly be the same. But most families find the path easier when they know for sure what they're dealing with.

- **Respect what the person having symptoms might be feeling**. Denial is a powerful self-protective emotion. That's why many people prefer to ignore bothersome symptoms rather than risk having to confront a problem. Some people fear the stigma that Alzheimer's still carries, especially in some cultures.

  Fear feeds denial. It's helpful to reassure: You're safe and you're with me, no matter what. We'll figure it out.

  Try realism framed in a positive way: "There are many treatable causes of memory loss and other cognitive symptoms besides Alzheimer's. If it is Alzheimer's, nothing will change overnight. You'll still be the same person who walked into the doctor's office. But now you'll know what you're up against and can do something about it."

- **Pursue diagnosis on a timetable that makes sense**. If you're still met with resistance, tread lightly. While you're smart to stick with your resolve to have concerns checked out, you have to realize that you might need to slow down. Badgering or bickering about it tends to lead to more resistance. It's best to move forward with compassion. The reality is that how you proceed from day to day isn't likely to change much whether you have a confirmed diagnosis of Alzheimer's or not.

  There's usually no rush. As symptoms progress, the person may be more willing to see a doctor, or a regular exam will come up for another reason. You can call in your concerns in advance of the appointment.

- **Create a record**. It's almost always family members, more than physicians, who spot the first signs of Alzheimer's disease. Write down examples of what you and others are seeing. You'll be better able to notice patterns or changes in the frequency of certain behaviors than you would by keeping a mental record. Include the dates of concerning events. This evidence is incredibly useful when you speak with medical professionals and may help when discussing the topic with family and friends.

Write down:

- Examples of memory loss

- Specific safety incidents (car accident, falls, getting lost, stove burners left on, etc.)

- Other unusual personality shifts or behaviors (incontinence, out-of-character outbursts, mood swings, etc.)

The key is change: anything that's different for that person. Be sure to note when you first noticed a particular change in behavior, physical ability, or mental ability (or about how long the change has been occurring); how frequently it occurs; if it has worsened; and how unlike the person it is.

This same notebook can also serve as your "playbook" throughout your family's journey, a central source of all the information that will be needed not only to make a diagnosis but to formulate an ongoing care plan. Having all the information you need in one place can be a valuable shortcut for families.

What else to record:

- Any current and past medical problems and conditions

- Current medications and their dosages

- Other family members' histories of illnesses (especially diabetes, heart disease, and Alzheimer's disease and other types of dementia)

- Contact information for doctors and pharmacists

- A record of who has been consulted and when

- While you're dealing with resistance, invest a little time in getting more familiar with the disease. Having a basic understanding allows you to ask doctors more informed questions and recognize the signs to watch for.

Creative solutions:

- **Try a "side door" approach to getting the person to a doctor**. Make it about you: "I know you feel perfectly healthy, but I've heard everyone over 60 should see the doctor once a year to check the heart and blood sugar, and you'll help me sleep better if you do that." If you're worried about one parent, get both parents to agree to "get checked out."

- **Try a third-party approach**. Sometimes spouses or parents won't listen to us but will willingly follow the suggestions of a friend, clergyperson, or other relative with more distance and less emotional history.

- **Register your concerns with your loved one's primary care doctor**. You can do this even if you don't have legal access to her health records. The doctor can't release information to you without the patient's consent, but you can share information or concerns. Ideally, time your call for just before a scheduled exam.

Really creative solutions:

- **Appeal to pride**. Some people might be persuaded to consult a specialist if you highlight something truly "special" about it to them: "This clinic is where so-and-so celebrity / local elites all go." Lisa P. Gwyther and Dr. Murali Doraiswamy, in their *Alzheimer's Action Plan*, note that this tactic got one woman to see a specialist with a "Christian medical practice," and another man agreed to a certain institution because it had once "saved my father's life." A former academic might be persuaded by an article about the doctor or clinic you have in mind.

- **Try a little white lie**: "The insurance company says you have to have a physical."

- **Try getting your loved one to the doctor for an entirely different reason**—a follow-up exam for a chronic condition, an unrelated symptom. Beforehand, express your concerns about memory, cognition, and other issues so the doctor is on alert. In the absence of another reason for an exam, consider asking the doctor about inviting your relative in for a checkup on some other pretext (a flu shot, an overdue preventative test). Some may agree to this in order to check out your concerns.

- **Look into house calls**. Some physicians, gerontologists, and geriatric care managers are among those who provide them and can do an initial assessment.

- **Look into a free screening**. The Alzheimer's Foundation of America sponsors a National Memory Screening Program, which offers confidential screenings by healthcare professionals. This may appeal to the budget-minded. (See "Resources.")

- **Pitch prevention, without mentioning your suspicions**: "I hear there's a lot we can do now to avoid Alzheimer's and memory problems. Let's find out what we can both do." Or, "Let's all go to get a baseline screening about how our brains are working now—then we can go have lunch after."

o o o

Rebuffs Your Assistance

"Certain subjects in our house were just taboo," recalls Kate. "And as my parents got older, #1 was the subject of their getting older. It just wasn't mentioned."

This drove Kate's husband, Dave, crazy. In his family, everybody talked about everything. His widowed mother was very open to Dave and his brothers taking care of her lawn, her house, and her finances.

Not so Kate's father. By the time his wife died, the house was already in disrepair. Two family inheritances had left the attics and hallways of the old house cluttered with extra furniture. He didn't cook much, either—which Kate secretly thought of as a blessing because she was afraid he might start a fire (even as she worried about his diet). He clearly needed help, but he carried on as if he were still 60 and hale, and besides, he said, it was "none of her damn beeswax."

"You have to do something!" Dave would say after each visit or crisis.

To which Kate would always say, "Yeah, but what? How?"

WHY it happens:

To allow help is to admit you need help. The number-one reason older adults often refuse assistance is fear of losing control. (It's number two and three and four, too.) Maintaining control is one of the driving needs of an older adult from the perspective of human development, says geriatric psychology and communication expert David Solie. "Each day, they feel losses—of strength, health, peers, and authority—that are staggering," he writes in his insightful book, *How to Say It to Seniors.*

Other factors that may contribute:

- *Pride and dignity.* Cooking, maintaining a home, or other aspects of self-care are points of pride for many. They see any intimation that they're no longer up to the task as insulting.

- *Stoicism.* Some people adapt to their "lot" in life, whatever it is. They had tough times before and see their current challenges as tough times to weather again.

- *Fractious relationships.* Resistance can be higher when there's suspicion (founded or not) of a family member's motives, such as concerns over money or a history of discord. Someone who doesn't believe you have his best interests at heart will balk.

- *Lack of insight.* In the early stages of Alzheimer's, your loved one may recognize that he's not managing as well but resist help. As the disease progresses beyond a certain point, he'll eventually lack the ability to even recognize that there's a problem.

The problem of a parent refusing help is among the most common and frustrating adult children encounter. Inserting yourself into someone's life is a worthy goal when you're doing it for his or her benefit. But parents don't always see it that way. They're driven by a need to be in control, and we're driven by a need to solve problems, get things done, tick items off a to-do list, and move forward. That disconnect can be crazy-making for both sides.

Someone with dementia is still a person with free will and preferences that deserve to be respected—at least up to the point when safety becomes an issue.

Knowing when you've reached that point, though, is never easy.

Early on, people can often continue to live independently if with an ever-increasing need for support. That's when it's important to tread carefully and compassionately, while exploring creative strategies for providing any necessary help. At the same time, the need to constantly monitor the environment to keep loved ones safe from their own limitations and from external threats grows almost daily. Everything from financial scammers and getting lost to malnourishment when they can no longer cook becomes a threat. We also have a moral duty to keep those around them safe—from being run down by poor driving or burned out of their apartment building because someone forgot to turn off a burner. This part of the journey can be a tricky dance, depending on the tone of your relationship and your loved one's personality, among other factors.

Eventually, everyone with dementia, if they live long enough, will need help in most areas of life. It becomes unsafe or impossible to do almost anything without supervision or help. If you're not at that point yet, it will come. That's when the tricky dance can become downright unpleasant, because you have to assert yourself in ways that may feel unnatural or unkind. And it can be hard to know when you've shifted from one phase to the next, because there's generally a long gray zone in the middle.

TRY this:

In the beginning...

- **Understand what "no" means**. Solie points out that knee-jerk refusals often come from the older person's compelling need to maintain control. It's a natural response to the conflicts they're feeling: coping with so many losses and threats, as well as to anyone (family caregivers included) trying to meddle and create more changes. Having empathy for this perspective can guide your communication. Let your loved one know that you get where he's coming from.

- **Listen more than act, at first**. Your goal is to help, not fight about the need for help. Invest time nurturing a relationship on a neutral, rather than adversarial, track. Spend time together not with the aim of nagging or saying what you think should be done but just relaxing and listening. Reassure that you care about his perspective. You'll be able to achieve more if he doesn't feel like you're "taking over" or "intruding."

- **Carefully research solutions before bringing them up**. Once you voice the problem, you'll need to be part of the solution. What resources are available in your community? Call the local Area Agency on Aging, which is a great starting point that will direct you to programs and services for specific needs. Your local Alzheimer's Association chapter may also have a list of services. If the problem is driving, look into alternate ways he could get around, such as paratransit services, Uber or Lyft, relatives pitching in to drive. If the problem is home repair, who can do it? If you need a personal care aide, what are the reputable services in town? Should you hire from them or try to find someone independently, which is usually cheaper but not regulated? Ask friends and colleagues. If you work for a large company, ask your human resources department for ideas.

- **Talk about the need for help only when the person is relaxed and in a good mood**. Consider whether you're the best messenger. Maybe a discussion about help would be more effective coming from the looked-up-to eldest sibling, an old family friend, or a trusted doctor.

- **Frame your ideas in positive terms**: "I used to think grab bars were ugly things, but I was reading up on what's called universal design, and now they're this trendy thing everyone wants and might help improve the value of the house." Or, "This program at the center is free if you're over 65—that's why Carol's mom and her friends all started going."

- **Instead of making suggestions, ask questions**: "I know you don't want to move, but how do you think we should handle upkeep on the house now that the doctor says you can't go up ladders?" "What do you want to do with all this extra stuff in the house?" "What's the most difficult part of living alone for you?"

  Try to listen for an underlying reason behind resistance that you might be able to address: concern about money or dislike of something new, for example.

- **Keep focused on the solution and the benefits**. "If someone helps with cleaning, I'll have more time to take you to lunch and the salon." "When your meals are brought to you, I won't have to worry as much, and you'll get your energy back."

- **Watch your language**. Some people bristle at certain words, like "help." Try words like maid service if "cleaners" offends, or car service instead of "somebody to drive you around."

- **Propose "temporary" solutions**: "Why don't you try this for a couple of months and see how it goes for you?" "The firm offers a trial service for a month. The first visit is free, so what's to lose?" One caregiver persuaded her parents to have a geriatric care manager (who she referred to as a life coach) drop by daily while she was out of town. Her parents enjoyed the help so much that the arrangement continued after the daughter's business trip ended.

- **Do what you can to prevent possible problems**. Often there are things you can do without permission or awareness that can extend the person's ability to live independently. You can turn down the temperature of the hot water to avoid accidental scalding, for example, or stop magazine subscriptions that pile up unread and get tripped over. Offer to automate bill pay.

Creative solutions:

- **Mask the purpose of the help**. Caregivers have hit on many clever strategies to bring in help, based on the quirks of their loved one and the needs of the situation. To help keep an eye on her mother across the country, for example, attorney and consumer advocate Barbara Kate Repa enlisted local friends who stopped by on pretexts. One friend asked Repa's mother to save the newspaper for her because she didn't subscribe. Every day or so she'd drop by to collect them. Another friend asked for knitting lessons. She also got her mom to accept Meals on Wheels services by telling her she was "rating" them for a work assignment and needed her help evaluating them.

- **Bestow a gift**. Your mother might not like the idea of a cook and maid because she's old and needs help, but she might get a kick out of a birthday gift for these services pitched as "pampering."

- **Find the right inroad**. Someone who never hired help but always follows clergy or medical advice might be open to someone coming in if recommended by the right person. Someone who grew up with household help might be more open to it, freeing you up to handle the caregiving chores.

- **Invoke others**. Some people are more accepting if they know it's what their peers do: "Jane's parents have a maid now" (even if that person is actually a personal aide).

- **Know your audience**. Some people are swayed by exclusivity or impressive credentials: "This is the best care manager in town, Mom." "It usually takes six months to get an appointment with this lawyer, but she had a cancellation and can see you next week."

- **Keep in mind that it's hard to force anybody to do anything**. You may have to live with decisions or living situations you're not thrilled with and wait for the proverbial other shoe to drop. This can be agonizing, especially as the effects of dementia begin to take hold. You may be only able to do what you can preventatively, until things reach the point where finances, health, or physical safety are in jeopardy.

When safety is at risk...

Sometimes families successfully get together and intervene to protect a loved one in danger. This tends to work better with a married couple. At first both refuse help, but as the dementia worsens, the well spouse capitulates and agrees that a new situation demands changes. A single older parent may decline to the point where family members are simply able to take on more and more, with less and less resistance.

What if these options don't pan out? You have plenty of company. Many families are driven to wit's end over this issue. If help is refused and your loved one continues to act in irresponsible or dangerous ways, you may have to resort to the "big gun" of the law.

- If he or she has previously assigned powers of attorney for health care and finances, it may be time to invoke those documents. Often this is a matter of a doctor or designated others declaring that the person can't make the relevant decisions.

- If you don't already have legal authority, you may need to seek adult guardianship, a more complex maneuver. It's also known as "conservatorship" in some states. You'll have to petition a judge to declare that the person is unable to make major decisions for himself and has made no previous documentation for what should happen in this event. The same person, or two different people, might be assigned to manage health decisions and financial-legal decisions.

  The benefits are huge: Your family gets clarity in a dangerous and disintegrating situation about how to safeguard your loved one.

  Unfortunately, guardianship is an expensive and often fraught process. You have to hire a lawyer and go before a judge. If the family member still has some awareness (or good days and bad, where it comes and goes), he may feel humiliated or emotionally manipulated by the very family members who are trying to save him.

  When families disagree over who should handle decision-making, a mediator may also need to be involved. If you go this route, look for an attorney who specializes in elder law, usually family attorneys. (Search elder mediation.) You'll need someone experienced to walk you through the nuances and help you prepare a case. You may have heard that it's difficult to obtain adult guardianship, but in cases of Alzheimer's, it tends to be much easier to prove the need for this step.

To help you cope:

- **Try not to get caught up in thoughts like these**: "I don't want to hurt her feelings." "That would be insulting to her dignity." "She'll hate me if I do that." "That's just not done in our family." Such beliefs might be true in a perfect world, but once your loved one has advancing dementia, you're in Alzheimer's world. To keep someone safe, the need for safety has to outweigh convention, pride, and hurt feelings. It's hard, but it's true.

- **Don't take these clashes personally**. It's not about you, the wisdom of your insights, the kindness of your heart, or the brilliance of your solutions. Recalcitrance has everything to do, instead, with your loved one's motivations and place in life. You might not get anywhere faster by taking your emotions out of the equation, but you'll get there with fewer hurt feelings.

o o o

BEHAVIOR CHALLENGES

Aggression (Acting Hostile or Violent)

"Carl didn't have a mean bone in his body," his widow, Esther, recalls. "He was as gentle as you can imagine helping birth a stuck foal or holding a grandbaby or oh, just anything."

Alzheimer's disease changed Carl. Though never a big talker, he became taciturn and sometimes even rude. He'd say curt, cutting things to visitors. He'd turn and leave the room on them. To Esther, his wife of 57 years, he was mostly docile and polite. Until the "ham sandwich incident," that is.

"I was serving him a late lunch one afternoon because we'd been out at the market," she says. "And when I put the ham sandwich down in front of him, he looked at it like he didn't know what it was, so I told him. 'I don't like ham! You know that!' he bellowed at me. I was so surprised.

"'Why Carl, of course you do,' I told him, easy as you please. And he reached up and slapped me across the face!" Esther is as astonished today, telling that story, as she was four years ago when it happened. "He'd never raised a hand to me for the world!"

That day marked a turning point. Carl continued to react with a raised hand whenever he didn't like something or didn't want to do it. Sometimes he grabbed her by the arm and clenched it. Esther, a petite woman, grew afraid. She hid Carl's rough behavior from her son until he saw it firsthand and made the connection to the bruises his mother had been making excuses for. They were investigating nursing homes when Carl died of a stroke.

WHY it happens:

Lashing out is usually a result of both brain changes and environmental factors. It's extremely upsetting, and sometimes dangerous, for family members.

The causes include:

- *Personality changes rooted in mental changes.* When someone with dementia becomes increasingly paranoid, frightened, or angry, he's more prone to explosive behavior.

- *Loss of inhibition and social appropriateness.* When angry impulses are tripped, self-control and self-censoring don't work the way they do in a healthy person.

- *A situation that's frightening or threatening.* This is related to brain changes. When he can't understand what the person helping him bathe is doing, for example (because he's lost the ability to recognize that he's dirty or what shower gel is) he may feel scared or violated. All kinds of circumstances can be misinterpreted. Being left alone for five minutes can feel like five hours when someone with dementia has lost the ability to track time, for example.

- *A situation that makes your loved one feel insecure or uncomfortable.* In addition to misperceptions, environmental realities can become irritating—too much noise, an unfamiliar new aide.

- *An underlying illness or physical problem.* Untreated pain can be expressed in violence by someone lacking the ability to recognize or describe that pain. In some people, the condition called delirium can lead to aggressive behaviors. An infection, sleep deprivation, dehydration, or some other stressor can bring on delirium. [See "Confusion That Suddenly Worsens (Delirium)" in the section on Health Challenges later in this chapter.] In Carl's case, for example, the aggression was a new behavior that came on suddenly, rather than a pattern of behaviors over time—a red flag for a physical cause.

- *An undetermined cause.* Whatever the trigger, the person reacts in a rough, hostile, or even violent way: hitting, scratching, biting, pushing, slamming doors, throwing things, screaming, insulting, or resisting any attempt at assistance.

These behaviors are usually directed toward the hands-on helper but may also be done to others in the household, animals, or objects.

It's easy to misread the hostility and violence of someone with dementia as a lack of gratitude, rudeness, or meanness. Though those things may seem true on the surface, it's important to remember that the aggression is telling you something quite different. Lacking the ability to fully process what's happening or express feelings of discomfort well, these behaviors are a physical expression of mood: "I'm upset." "I'm angry." "I'm scared." "I'm so confused." "I feel overwhelmed and out of control."

TRY this:

In the moment:

- **Hard as this can be, try not to take aggression personally and avoid reacting in kind**. Raising your voice in response, threatening, or acting more forcefully can cause aggression to escalate. Your goal is the opposite: to reassure.

- **Back off, rather than moving in to physically restrain**. Not only might you get hurt if you try to subdue the aggressive person, but you'll cause him to fight harder. Backing off is defensive, protective—and, ultimately, ends the episode quicker.

- **Stop doing whatever was happening at the moment**. If you were trying to help the person toilet or dress, withdraw. Give yourselves both a moment to calm down. If possible, don't return to that task at all until you sense the time is right.

- **Stick to a calm response and a pleasant expression**. Even a smile—though that won't be your natural first response and may seem inappropriate—is helpful because body language is powerful and is understood more quickly than words, especially when someone is acting on a primal level. An angry response will be mirrored back.

- **Offer a mild or soothing verbal response**: "Everything's all right now." "Can I help you with something?" "I'm sorry you're upset." "Let's watch the birds out the window until you feel better."

- **Step out of the room for a few minutes if you need a moment to collect yourself**. Better that objects are thrown or furniture is overturned than you risk injury yourself.

- **When the outburst and its aftermath are over, avoid returning to the same activity**. Try something pleasant or distracting—a root beer float, sitting on the porch, listening to some favorite music. Wait to repeat the fraught activity until he's in a calmer frame of mind. Try to avoid the exact thing you were doing at the time of the incident and do it in a slightly changed way (different tool, different approach, different order, different person) to avoid an instant replay.

Tip: **"Figure out an arsenal of soothers that are things your person usually softens to. For us it's ice cream, singing, and a stuffed dog. Hard to be hostile when you're petting your favorite stuffed puppy." —R.E.**

To minimize further episodes:

- **Look for changes in the environment to see if you can identify what set off the aggression**: Has a busy day left him tired? Is he sick or in pain? Is there a new helper who does things differently? Focus on what might be new or different. Beware of new medications. They can intensify aggression, either as a side effect or as an interaction with other meds. Take steps to avoid "trigger situations" once you've identified them.

- **Reinforce routines and consistency**. Everything you can do to create a secure, predictable environment can help. But know, too, that you can do everything right, and a confused mind may still imagine injustice or fear, or feel pain.

- **See if you can detect any physical changes that indicate a blow-up is building**. They vary by person, but clues might include a reddening face, a quavering or raised voice, and shaking hands. Stopping what you're doing (or changing the environment) and switching to something more calming can help avert an outburst.

- **Report dangerous behaviors to his or her doctor**. It's important to rule out underlying medical problems—not only delirium but also chronic pain or illnesses such as depression or other mental conditions that can be treated with medication. Sometimes medications such as anti-anxiety drugs or anti-depressants are used to control aggression. So are anti-psychotics, although these raise the risk of stroke and death, and there's a strong shift away from their use for treating Alzheimer's patients. Every case should be assessed individually, weighing benefits against risks.

- **Get some targeted training**. Consider asking the doctor, a support group, the local Alzheimer's Association, or another outlet about training tips to deal with aggression and dementia (or difficult behaviors generally).

- **Remove all firearms from the home**. Forty percent of veterans with dementia have them, reports the VA. Even if the person who has dementia has always used them responsibly in the past, or doesn't know how to use them because they belong to someone else, Alzheimer's changes everything. Anger, disinhibition, despondency, and cloudy thinking have merged in tragic ways. You can call your local sheriff's department or other law enforcement to retrieve the gun for you. The Alzheimer's Association notes that they may want to see a statement of diagnosis from the person's doctor. Or ask a family member to store it. If the person asks about a missing gun, you can try saying that a friend has "borrowed" it or it's been sent for a professional cleaning ("as a gift") or is out for repair. Alternately, you can have the gun made inoperable, but it's really safest to leave nothing to chance.

- **Know that aggressive tendencies often worsen**. If you ever don't feel safe, it may be time to consider out-of-home placement. Sadly, smaller spouses with a large mate who tends to lash out suddenly sometimes find this to be the case due to the sheer size disparity.

To help you cope:

- **Don't be surprised when the person later acts (after a hostile incident) as if nothing happened**. He probably doesn't remember the outbursts. But if you persist in a grudging, angry mood—it's a natural impulse to want to hold hostile acts against the perpetrator—he won't understand why and may parrot back your attitude. With dementia, he's not "acting innocent" afterward to manipulate you. That's why it's best to simply attribute the behavior to the disease and move on—provided, of course, that you protect yourself.

- **Find outlets for your own feelings**. You'll be upset. You'll want to react. That's only natural—and you should. It's just counterproductive for these reactions to be directed at the person with dementia. Far better to get your feelings out another way instead of lashing back or keeping them bottled up, where they can endanger your heart health and immune system. Punch pillows. Walk up and down stairs quickly. Have a friend or two on speed dial. Set up a dartboard in your bedroom. Write in a diary. But please, pick healthy outlets. Turning to drugs or alcohol won't do you or your loved one much good in the long run.

- **Know that it's common to feel you're living with a stranger, once aggression enters the picture**. This is especially true if a beloved person never showed such tendencies before. This can be a sad and isolating feeling, especially for spousal caregivers. Do reach out to a support group or online support network for the extra positive reinforcement you need.

o o o

Agitation and Meltdowns

We grew to know when my father-in-law was upset about something because he began to empty his room: bins of papers, clothes on hangers, the wastebasket filled with toiletries, even boxes of Depends. Never mind that he needed a walker. Somehow he'd balance a load on top of it and make his way to the driveway. There, he'd set down the stuff and head back across the rear patio to fetch more. After spending a couple of hours shuffling back and forth, to and fro, a burst of energy unlike his usual mode, he'd sit on a little ledge next to the pile and mutter. "Where is she (or he)?" Someone—variously an imaginary wife, friend, or taxi driver— was bringing "the Buick" around to pick him up, he'd say.

Worked up to begin with, he got even madder as he waited, since no one ever actually was coming. Once he somehow climbed into my Subaru and impatiently honked the horn over and over until we coaxed him out.

A friend's mother expressed agitation in an even more kinetic way. She often sat in a chair rocking, pulling yarn from a skein and loosely balling it, kneading it in her hands. Especially in the evening, this activity seemed to soothe her. But at other times, she'd begin to rock harder and faster. Her hand motions grew wilder and she shouted random, often unintelligible, things.

Her grandchildren learned to steer clear of Nana when she was like this. It's scary, they said. —P.S.S.

WHY it happens:

Restlessness and mood swings may show up as nervous tics of repetitive actions or just a lot of twitchy, fidgety energy. Sometimes these behaviors simmer on low, other times they build and boil over. The person with dementia may seem to fly off the handle in a way that's out of proportion to the situation.

Sometimes agitation erupts into a catastrophic reaction—a fancy way of saying meltdown.

Agitation may also take the form of specific behaviors such as pacing, rummaging, cursing, screaming, and aggression. Agitation may also worsen late in the day (sundowning).

The main causes include:

- *A psychiatric issue.* Agitation is more common in a dementia personality type that's paranoid, frightened, or angry. Less often, you see it in someone who's anxious or depressed. If you're seeing hallucinations and false beliefs, you may also see these agitated outbursts.

- *A physical problem.* When it's a new or sudden behavior, agitation can be a sign of delirium, which is caused by an underlying stressor to the body, such as infection or dehydration, or a reaction to a medication. This could be a new problem or a flare-up of a chronic disease. Disrupted sleep and pain can also lead to increased agitation, and being hungry or tired can intensify the response.

- *Stress from changes in the environment.* Examples include a new caregiving aide, a disrupted routine, crowds, too much noise, or a long wait at a busy doctor or dentist's office.

- *A departure from routine or what's expected.* Some people with dementia are highly anxious. A change in schedule (meals that are late) or a caregiver who's out of sight (in the basement doing laundry or off at work) can set off a meltdown out of proportion to the incident itself.

- *Being rushed* or feeling pressured in any way.

- *Boredom*, lack of constructive activity, being left alone.

TRY this:

- **Tell the doctor when agitation is a sudden, recent change**. Get a medical exam to rule out a physical cause.

- **Don't respond in kind**. It's critical to remain low-key to avoid revving up an agitated reaction further. Use a soothing, even voice to reassure: "You're all right. I'm right here. Nothing to worry about."

- **Don't bother to scold or criticize someone who's behaving inappropriately**. This isn't about what's "right." It's about getting back to calm.

- **Give the person space to vent or act up if it seems harmless**. Some people get worked up until they tire, then sleep and seem fine. Your main goals should be to calm and keep the person safe. In my father-in-law's case, we'd offer him food in hopes of distracting him (which he refused if he was really worked up) but otherwise let him continue, and commiserated with him about being stood up. That seemed to calm him and felt kinder than restraining or contradicting him by hauling everything back in his room. (Eventually, we found a solution he accepted: We stored all the non-essentials he emptied from his room out of sight, until he'd need them—because "it was about to rain," we told him.)

- **Avoid sudden movements**. It can be a natural response to want to restrain or cordon off someone who's having a meltdown. But those actions can be perceived as a threat, adding a bellow's breath to the fire.

To avoid agitated responses:

- **Arrange your lives around a routine**. Predictability is reassuring and can help ward off agitated responses.

- **Do everything you can to keep daily life calm**. Along with routine, this means keeping noise levels down (including a blaring TV or radio) and keeping lights bright but soft (lower or close shades when sunlight creates glare).

- **Avoid activities that cause undue frustration**. You don't want to do everything for the person, which can lead to boredom, but you do want to aim for a sweet spot where he or she can enjoy simple successes. Try encouraging creative expression (painting, singing, crafts), which can be a welcome outlet for someone whose capacity for verbal expression is giving them trouble. Also soothing: listening to music, driving in a car, or making something (such as helping you make cookies)—so long as you keep the focus on the process and off the performance or end result.

- **Try making available activities that channel nervous energy**. Popular examples: fidget spinners, stress balls, cards to shuffle, activity aprons or quilts (also called busy quilts or fidget blankets), crocheting (someone who knew how may still have the muscle memory to continue), or a junk drawer or toolbox to sort through.

- **Give yourself extra time for challenging activities**. Feeling pressured or rushed can feed agitation.

o o o

Can't Make Decisions

Every Sunday, Jack took his grandfather to church and out to brunch. He liked spending time with Pappy and it was a way to give his parents, with whom Pappy lived, a needed break. "Why don't you find a table while I wash my hands." he told his grandfather. They came here every week and usually sat by the windows. But when Jack exited the restroom, he was surprised to find Pappy still standing in the same spot.

He led him to their usual row of booths. "Look, they have both your favorites today, the maple waffles and the blueberry pancakes," Jack noted. When the waitress approached, Jack respectfully indicated his grandfather order first. "Well..." he said uncertainly. The waitress waited, pen poised. "Well, let's see," said Pappy.

"Maple waffles? Blueberry pancakes?" Jack prompted helpfully. "Or do you feel like eggs today?"

"Well..."

Finally Jack ordered first. Then it was back to Pappy, who still frowned at the menu. "How about the waffles? You like those," Jack finally suggested.

"Sure," said Pappy brightly. Waffles it was.

WHY it happens:

Decision-making involves remembering past preferences, weighing the pros and cons of the options, and assessing how you feel in the moment—mental calculations that a healthy brain can make instantly. But that seemingly simple ability to hold several ideas in mind at once and choose between them is a skill that dementia begins to erode even in the early stages of the disease.

For someone who has Alzheimer's, every decision, large or small—which table to choose in a restaurant, what to order, what to say or do next—can seem overwhelming, making the person feel frustrated and anxious.

They may be afraid of making what will be seen as the "wrong" choice. Or they simply might not remember what the options are.

TRY this:

- **Wait patiently for a reply rather than jumping in immediately**. Making the other person feel rushed can add to anxiety.

- **If you see that the person is having trouble after a short spell**—or if it's happened before—step in with a single suggestion or prompt: "Let's order the special." Or, "I'm having the tuna melt. You want one too?"

- **Limit choices as much as possible to relieve unneeded stress**. Especially eliminate open-ended choices. Avoid asking, "What do you want to eat?" or "What do you want to do today?" Better: "The special is spaghetti. Should we order that?" "Let's go to the park now."

- **Know that when you give several choices, the person will often simply parrot back the last thing you said**. So if you ask, "Do you want vanilla, strawberry, or chocolate ice cream?" the answer will likely be "chocolate." It can be helpful to offer up the last choice if you think it's what he prefers (or if that's easiest all around).

- **Simplify choices overall**: Avoid buffets. Stock fewer clothes in the dresser and closet. Guide selections when shopping, because even picking toothpaste involves dozens of options. Anticipate your loved one's preferences and find graceful ways to make choices for him.

- **Don't necessarily eliminate all choices**. Having the power to say "this" or "that" gives all of us a welcome sense of control over our environment. You could start from a place of simple options (say, between two items), but back off when even that's clearly proving more overwhelming than empowering.

o o o

Crying Jags (or Laughing Jags)

Millie's son can tell his mother is awake because the moaning cries rise up from her bed and crackle over the monitor to his room. She seems to wake up crying and often continues to moan, wail, and rock for hours. She pauses to eat or is sometimes distracted by the birds outside or her dog, but soon enough is wailing again.

WHY it happens:

There's often both an immediate reason for wailing and tears and a chronic one. Doctors call it "emotional lability" or emotional incontinence—an inability to manage emotional output. Less often, it's expressed as laughing jags.

In the immediate moment, the person feels a need to release emotion. The trigger can be anything: either specific (a perceived slight, a room that's too dark or too bright, too much noise) or, more often, broad (pain, boredom, loneliness, missing a deceased partner). For those who retain some awareness of their condition (or awareness that something's "not right" and life is a struggle), this knowledge alone can be enough to trigger tears.

One of two conditions usually underlies frequent crying:

1. *Clinical depression.* People with dementia are more prone than others to clinical depression for reasons that aren't fully understood.

2. *Pseudobulbar affect (PBA).* This brain disorder can be caused by Alzheimer's or other kinds of brain injury, such as a stroke or a head injury after a fall. The crying is not only socially inappropriate but often doesn't fit the circumstances (such as crying at a party). It's often mistaken for depression in someone with Alzheimer's. The National Stroke Association estimates that 1 million people may have PBA.

Crying jags aren't unusual in moderate or early severe-stage dementia. Some people cry or laugh intermittently for hours at a stretch—an indicator of depression. With PBA, the bouts tend to be shorter (a matter of minutes) but can go on all day.

TRY this:

- **Offer empathy**: "You sound so sad. Can I help?" If you ask, "What's wrong?" your loved one will probably not be able to articulate her feelings.

- **Provide physical support and affection**—hugs, shoulder pats or rubs, and so on. Someone with dementia who's depressed has a deep need for both verbal and physical reassurance. Say, "It's okay. You're safe with me. Everything's all right."

- **Mention the behavior to the doctor**. It's important to look for other symptoms of depression, but also bring up the possibility of pseudobulbar affect, since it's under-diagnosed in Alzheimer's. Both PBA and clinical depression are treatable even in someone with moderate-stage Alzheimer's. Unfortunately, both involve medication at a time in life when it's ideal to minimize medications, but depending on the severity of the behavior, treatment can make life more bearable for everyone.

Tip: "**We played a lot of slapstick old movies, like Charlie Chaplin, Abbott and Costello, Marx Brothers, and the Our Gang shows. When my mother was laughing, she didn't cry. It was like turning the spigot off for a while.**" —**B.J.E.**

To help you cope:

- **Know it's okay not to solve the problem**. When a baby or small child cries, we're wired to rush in to fix it. But the crying jags of Alzheimer's can't always be fixed. Sometimes, you just have to endure them. Follow the steps above, and take solace that you've done all you can to be reassuring and to address the problem medically.

o o o

Follows You Everywhere (Shadowing)

When Stan gets up from his living room lounger to get some coffee, so does Stella, his wife of 51 years. "I'll bring it to you," he says.

"Okay," says Stella. But she follows him anyway. She follows him upstairs and downstairs, inside and outside. Lately, when he uses the bathroom, she's standing right outside the door waiting for him when he comes out.

WHY it happens:

A trusted family member can be a strong source of security and reassurance to someone with Alzheimer's—a kind of anchor in her increasingly confused world. You represent safety and steadfastness. You help her avoid embarrassment or frustration. In addition to the reassurance of your presence, she might be dependent on your knowledge and answers. Shadowing can increase if the person is bored.

For all these reasons, many people with dementia want to keep their primary caregiver in their direct line of vision at all times. They become almost your "shadow."

Some caregivers think shadowing happens because their loved one doesn't trust them, and it can certainly feel that way. But it's not about you (even if they say so). It's the disease feeding fear and anxiety about disorienting experiences.

TRY this:

- **Reinforce efforts to keep to a predictable household routine**. Eating, resting, exercising, and leaving the house in the same order and at about the same times every day contribute to a feeling of security.

- **See if you can identify a pattern**: Does shadowing increase at a particular time of day? When certain people are around?

- **Try saying something reassuring** ("Hello, dear"), rather than showing annoyance or impatience. For stability's sake, it's important that you continue to be a calm social refuge.

- **Make sure your loved one has activities that absorb her**. It's okay if they're repeats of things you just did yesterday or earlier in the day, like raking leaves or folding towels, as long as she seems into it.

- **Develop a handful of reassuring phrases**: "It's a beautiful, day, Sweetheart." "You look wonderful today; I love you." Repetition of certain phrases works well for many.

- **Use music to soothe**. Try preparing a calming or reassuring playlist that your loved one can sit and listen to through headphones. (Headphones aren't necessary, but they can be handy if you get tired of listening to certain tracks over and over.)

- **Try not to go out of sight for long periods of time**. People with dementia can't track time well. Five minutes might seem like an hour. If you must be out of the room for a while (such as to shower or to do laundry in a basement), check in verbally every few minutes.

- **Set a timer when you take a shower or have a similar task**. Simply say, "When the bell dings, I'll be done." Use a timer that makes a reassuring ticking sound and place it where the person can watch it. When you return, say, "See, I came back just like I said I would when the timer dinged."

Tip: **"I used a baby monitor when I had to leave the room. I would keep talking into it so my mom could hear my voice. I'd tell her where I was and that I'd be right back."** **—J.G.**

To help you cope:

- **Be sure to arrange regular respite for yourself**. Ideally, it should be every day or at least every other day or so—even if only for an hour or two while you go for a walk or have a cup of coffee with a friend. Don't think that because your loved one is so dependent on you that your constant presence is an absolute necessity. She'll manage well enough under someone else's temporary attentive care. What's more, the distractions of a day program (or a new presence) can help ease the person's boredom, which contributes to shadowing.

- **Know that even when you love the person with dementia dearly**, even when you've spent a lifetime together, shadowing is different. It can become claustrophobic and stressful. Humans need some privacy! Being able to have someone else spend short amounts of time with your loved one is critical for your mental health.

o o o

Hallucinates (Sees and Hears Things That Aren't There)

"Good morning," I said as I entered the kitchen.

My mother-in-law, in her mid-80s, smiled. "Did you see that grizzly bear in the yard?"

"No, where?" I asked in surprise and mild panic, looking out the kitchen window into her suburban New Jersey back yard.

"Last night! It was standing up, right over there! I called the police!"

"Last night?" I asked, confused. "Police?" She had gone to bed first, and it had been a peaceful evening.

"Oh, yes! A bunch of men came over with guns!"

As it happened, there was no police report of any such incident, no word of bears in the neighborhood—and, in fact, no bear.

This episode was surreal. But years later, my father-in-law (from my second marriage, not her husband) often saw, and interacted with, invisible "family." He had several imaginary wives, for example, whom he'd talk to for hours. Another time, he asked me to call "the little boys" to the lunch table and make them peanut butter sandwiches. Saddest was the time he asked for help finding "my little red-haired granddaughter," supposedly a 4-year-old who had just used the bathroom off his room and then disappeared. He looked and looked for her. Later I found him sitting on his bed with his head in his hands. "Oh, Paula," he cried. "Where could she have gone to? Oh, what will I tell her mother?"
—P.S.S.

WHY it happens:

Hallucinations—seeing, hearing, feeling, smelling, or even tasting things that aren't there—usually occur in the later stages of dementia due to brain changes and difficulty telling fantasy from reality.

A person may hear voices and even chat or argue with a long-dead relative. Another may feel like her hair is on fire or smell fire where there is none. Still another person might claim to see ants in her food. Any of these things seem absolutely real to the person with dementia. They may or may not be upsetting.

These perception changes can worsen in the evening. Triggers can include stress, unusual noise or light, or lack of sleep. Hearing or vision problems can intensify the misperception. (For example, my father-in-law—after his eyesight started failing—watched what he insisted was a nun standing outside next door, for hours. He finally urged me to go talk to her. She was a golf bag someone had stuck in a trashcan.)

Hallucinations can also be part of delirium, especially if they're sudden in onset, caused by an underlying stressor, such as an infection or pain. Some medications can also cause false perceptions.

Estimates range widely as to how common hallucinations are in people with Alzheimer's. Studies report anywhere from 10 to 60 percent of patients have some kind at some point. (Hallucinations are even more common in another type of dementia, Lewy Body.) And people with Alzheimer's who experience hallucinations are at increased risk for faster cognitive and functional decline, studies show.

TRY this:

- **Assess the impact of the hallucination**. You don't have to do much if it's not upsetting the person (not causing fear or agitation, for example) or leading to dangerous behavior (such as refusing to eat or leading her outdoors where she's prone to wandering off).

- **Avoid correcting her or trying to prove the illogic of the perception**. Realize that it seems quite real to her and that she can't be argued out of it.

- **Acknowledge the imaginary perception**. Comment in a way that's matter of fact and reassuring. A little white lie of agreement is okay here ("I'm glad to hear the police took care of it and everything is safe and back to normal. Do you want toast for breakfast?")

- **Use empathetic phrasing that plays back the person's feelings**: "That must have been scary." "I can see that you're not happy about that."

- **If the hallucination is upsetting, assure your loved one that you'll take care of it**. Remind her with words and a soothing hug that she's safe with you and everything will be all right. ("The little girl is safe now. Our neighbor found her and drove her home.")

- **Go along with what you reasonably can**. One woman put out leftovers for imaginary cats, and her daughter emptied the dishes when her mom napped. Another caregiver provided a flashlight for her dad to chase the "little people under my bed."

- **Distract with a pleasant experience, such as a favorite snack or a game of cards**. Play soothing music or introduce a change of scenery by moving to a different room or going outside.

- **See if you can make a connection to reality that might be triggering the hallucination**. For example, a shadow of moving branches might be perceived as an intruder. Sounds of a violent TV show might be mistaken for events happening in the room. The hum of an air conditioner may sound like voices. There isn't always a logical connection, but it's worth considering in case you can fix the problem easily—for example by turning on a light or turning off the TV.

- **Avoid reminding the person of the incident later or bring it up again**. Often the person hallucinating quickly forgets even a startling experience. (The rest of the household might be shaken up for a while!)

- **If hallucinations persist, it's a good idea to get a medical check-up** to rule out possible causes apart from dementia, such as a urinary tract infection, a bad medication reaction, or dehydration. Also consult with the doctor if hallucinations become disruptive and constant, such as interfering with sleep. Anti-psychotic medications may help, though they're considered a last line of defense.

To help you cope:

- **Remember that many hallucinations are harmless**, so always start by asking yourself: Is the problem here how the perception is affecting the person with dementia, such as disrupting sleep? Or is it that she's doing or saying things that are embarrassing or unnerving to you?

o o o

Delusions (False Ideas or Accusations)

"You hussy!" Leonard hissed at Lou, his wife of 53 years, when she entered the room.

"What did you call me?" she said, taken aback.

"I saw you, sneaking off with that gardener! I was watching you through the window! You didn't think I saw you, but I know all about your flirting and your running around!"

Gardener? Running around? Lou had never so much as looked at another man before. And they'd never had a gardener at their tiny suburban bungalow. "Stop talking nonsense!" she admonished. But Leonard only sneered at her more, until she burst into tears and had to leave the room.

Stepping onto the front porch for air, she realized that shortly before the tirade, she'd gone to the front yard to give the boy across the street some lemonade and some money. His mother had asked him to start cutting their lawn after noticing it getting shaggy. Leonard couldn't do it anymore, and Lou seldom had time herself. She'd been so grateful. How could Leonard think she was flirting with the kid? He was all of 13!

WHY it happens:

Because someone with dementia has lost the ability to reason and make accurate judgments, he may blame others for any confusion or difficulty he encounters. Things he can't make sense of leave him feeling anxious. Can't find his glasses? That aide stole them! Doesn't recognize a neighbor who's mowing his lawn for him? He must be the fella sneaking around with my wife!

Known as paranoid delusions, false accusations can take many forms. Among the most common irrational beliefs for people with dementia: accusing someone of stealing, accusing a spouse of adultery, believing the house is being invaded, claiming that family members have been replaced by impostors. Nearly one in three people with Alzheimer's have delusions, and the number is higher for those with frontotemporal dementia.

Delusions can happen at any stage of dementia but have been found to be most common in the moderate stage of disease, as the ability to distinguish reality erodes.

TRY this:

- **Skip trying to prove your innocence**, the way things really are, or berating the person for making an outrageous claim. The more you protest, the more fixed this belief often becomes.

- **Let the person talk**. Listen attentively and empathetically.

- **Ask questions that encourage details**: "What did she do?" "Where did they go?" "When did you notice your money was missing?" You're not doing this to collect evidence to "solve" the mystery. Rather, you're validating the person's perception—stepping into his world—by letting him share his thoughts, and you might get insight into the origin of the belief. For example, he might tell you that he knew his wife was replaced by an alien because her hair is different (and you know she just got a haircut). Avoid the one you're itching to ask most, though. You won't get any kind of useful answer to "Why?"

- **Avoid agreeing to a falsehood**. This is a situation where an agreeable white lie rarely pays off. You might make things worse ("You think she was stealing, too? I'm going to fire her right now!"). More likely, the person with dementia can't process what you're saying or may quickly forget and start the loop of accusing again.

- **Try defusing with humor**: "Sorry, you're stuck with me, dear. You know I've always been a one-man gal." Or, "I don't know why, but Mom insists you're mates for life."

- **Provide a simple solution, if you can**: "Look, here are your glasses." If certain objects go "missing" often, consider getting multiples of them.

- **Give lots of reassurance (without disputing the delusion)**: "It's safe now." "I love you." "We found your missing ring."

- **Keep a few dollars or an inactive credit card in the wallet of someone who often accuses others of stealing**. Often families remove these items for safety's sake, but that can have the unintended effect of upsetting the person, who fears he's been robbed because he's used to seeing money and cards in a wallet.

- **Distract**. Change the subject or move to another room. "Let's talk about this some more after we check the bird feeder." "Before we look for the missing candlesticks, let's get something to eat for energy."

- **Assure the accused that this is the disease talking**. Reassure that person that you value their presence and don't believe the falsity.

To help you cope:

- **Separate your feelings from the accusation**. Realize that these delusions have almost nothing to do with the quality of the relationship between the accuser and the accused. A beloved grandson might be accused of stealing money. The spouse in a long-happy marriage, who is a devoted caregiver, might get pegged as an adulterer.

- **Remind yourself that this is the disease talking, not the person**. Some delusions are so strange or upsetting to hear that it can be hard not to get annoyed, even when you're sure they're untrue. My father-in-law, for example, began to fabricate elaborate stories about the supposed wild affairs of his late wife (of 65 happy years) that were as comic in their details as their children knew them to be false. He told doctors. He told visitors. He'd rail on about the supposed adulterer, only to utterly forget about it when the man's wife sent a get-well card: "Gee, isn't that nice to hear from them!"

o o o

Hoarding, Hiding, and Clutter

Joanne's mother, Doris, had always been a bit disorganized and messy. Over the years, piles of papers seemed to grow on her desk, atop the kitchen counter, on the floor around her favorite lounge chair. At first, Joanne and her sister Beth just wrote the habit off as messiness. They got used to hearing Doris say, "I'm saving that to look at later," or "You never know when you might need it."

Eventually Doris began showing other symptoms of dementia, from forgetfulness to critical financial mistakes. Meanwhile the clutter grew. Doris began to save empty yogurt containers that she'd clean and stack on the windowsill. When her daughters asked why she was doing it, she'd brush them off: "Stay out of my kitchen!"

Doris, who was divorced, still lived alone. One day Beth visited and found empty yogurt containers—not all of them clean—on the windowsills of the dining room. She used the bathroom, and more yogurt cups lined the sill there. The house seemed full of more yogurts than her mother could have possibly eaten. Coming out of the bathroom with an armful to throw away, Doris had a fit. "Stop! Stop!" she cried, yanking her daughter's arm so the cups fell to the floor.

"Mom! These are dirty!" Beth explained. Doris hit her.

Beth retreated to her car and whipped out her cellphone. "Joanne," she said to her sister. "We've got to talk!"

WHY it happens:

Starting very early in the disease, people sometimes acquire multiples of certain types of objects to an unusual degree, beyond ordinary collecting. They may simply forget they've bought a certain kind of salad dressing, for example, and buy it every time they shop until suddenly there are a dozen identical bottles in the cupboard.

As judgment erodes, they may be reluctant to throw anything away—not only necessities but things that are no longer needed, even trash. Junk mail, empty tissue boxes, clothes, and other objects pile up.

They may hide objects, often in unusual or illogical places, to keep them safe. Conversely, some people keep things out where they're visible (toiletries on tabletops, clothes draped over stair railings) in order to keep them safe and not lose them.

About one in five people with Alzheimer's are thought to be true hoarders—those who obsessively collect and save objects to an extent that's potentially dangerous.

Unlike objects in a conventional collector's collection, these things may have no value (sentimental, monetary, or otherwise) and the practice can take over the person's life to a degree that's socially isolating or physically dangerous, such as clutter that represents a fire or tripping hazard.

Sometimes the objects are confined to one space. Sometimes there's clutter everywhere. Or objects might be hidden in unusual spots.

Common things people with Alzheimer's hoard, according to a study in the *American Journal of Geriatric Psychiatry*, include papers, daily necessities (such as toiletries), newspapers and magazines, plastic bags, old clothes, food, and garbage.

Causes of hoarding include:

- *An obsessive-compulsive disorder* that may have existed separately from the dementia. (People who were prone to clutter before dementia tend to get worse.)

- *Cognitive changes*. The person can no longer distinguish between what's worth saving and what isn't and can't make decisions. Memory loss may lead to a habit of misplacing objects and forgetting where they're stored.

- *Boredom* or lack of healthier stimulation.

- *Anxiety*. Fearing loss (or expressing loss), the person gets security from setting aside random objects. Hoarding is related to rummaging, as the person later searches for the objects and the mere act of touching them provides security.

TRY this:

- **When the person is asleep, thin the collection**. Leave several items, so it doesn't feel completely decimated yet is safer and more manageable. Getting rid of everything at once can be distressing and counterproductive. Throw away food items that aren't safe to save. Whatever you throw away should be removed from the home completely—not placed in the garbage or even the trashcan at the end of the driveway, where it can be searched for and retrieved.

- **Repeat clean-ups regularly**. Without ongoing help, the clutter will quickly return.

- **If asked where items have gone**, offer an explanation that the hoarder may respond to positively: You donated them to a family in need. You sent them out for cleaning.

- **Try making a visual record**. Some hoarders settle for a collection of photos of their collection. This works best for, say, a longtime doll collector or tool collector whose habit has gone haywire, rather than someone who compulsively saves everything.

- **Don't bother providing additional space or equipment for organizing the clutter**. Buying extra tables, baskets, and bins won't help. The problem is that the person can no longer organize. Extra space will only result in extra clutter.

- **Check preferred hiding spots regularly**. Many people develop certain quirky "go to" spots to hide things: kitchen canisters (for trash, rather than sugar and flour), certain drawers, under mattresses, laundry hampers, underused closets, in the bushes outside.

- **If you see the person rummaging around**, suggest these go-to hiding places. Even these favorite spots may be forgotten!

- **Plug up the sources of the incoming stuff, if you can**. Cancel newspaper or magazine subscriptions, block home shopping channels, close credit-card accounts.

See also in this chapter: "Rummaging"

o o o

Phones Over and Over

"It's Mom. When are you coming over?"

"Mom, I came by this morning. I'm at work now."

"Oh....sure...are you coming by later? I need you to look at my toaster."

"Yes, Mom, you already called me twice about that."

Tony's mother, Flora, lives alone ten minutes from his house. Even though he stops by before and after work, she's begun to call him increasingly often during the day and in the evening.

"It's Mom. Turn on channel 20. It's the funniest thing!"

"I can't, Mom, I'm at work."

"Oh, okay. Then why did you call me?"

WHY it happens:

The telephone is a kind of umbilical cord for your loved one representing security. Pick it up, and there you are. When feeling insecure, lonely, scared, or simply when thinking of you, your loved one places a call. Worsening memory makes her unable to remember that she called earlier (once, twice, a dozen times).

Familiar, long-dialed numbers—yours, the doctor's office, a friend's—tend to be called most often. A single-button speed-dial system makes it especially easy to call those individuals.

Some people dial 911 repeatedly to get a live human to talk to (not about an emergency), maybe because "911" is a deeply ingrained number.

Or calling becomes a behavioral tic, a form of repetitive behavior.

Be aware that not being able to use the phone properly—whether from overuse or avoidance—is a sign that someone who lives alone can't dial emergency services or 911 as needed, a red flag for being unable to live independently.

Other common phone problems:

She can't find and pick up the phone.

WHY: A cellphone might be confused for a TV remote or other gadget. Impaired thinking makes her unable to connect the ring with the need to pick it up. Or she may pick it up but not press the right button to activate a call. Some people who were older at the dawn of iPhones fail to "see" them as phones no matter how many times you show how it works.

She answers the phone but doesn't speak.

WHY: She doesn't recognize the disembodied voice. Or she has bad hearing on top of the dementia and can't hear it.

She answers the phone but doesn't take a message.

WHY: She may think she'll remember (but never does). Or she lacks the wherewithal to get a pen and go through the motions of writing down what's said.

TRY this:

The right solution depends on your specific situation, but these ideas may help:

- **Screen calls**. Switch to a phone with number recognition display (caller ID) or set a specific ring tone for your loved one, so you can decide which calls to answer. Especially at night, let the message go to voicemail and decide whether it's a crisis. The person may grow frustrated by not hearing your actual voice and begin to call less (although others will call more often).

- **If you live in the same house, cancel the landline and use only your cellphone**. That way, the person with dementia can't call out if she's a repetitive caller. Or place landlines only in the rooms where the person doesn't go, such as your bedroom and the basement.

- **Claim you're making the switch to "save money."** It's an appeal that works for many Depression-era children.

- **Avoid having calls come into the home**. Use call forwarding to send home calls to your cellphone.

- **Turn down ringers**. Not hearing the phone ring may make it less top-of-mind.

- **For people with early stage disease**: Look into easy-to-use models that have visual cue buttons to easily identify family members or emergency help. Another option, for those who call often: dial-less phones that receive calls but don't permit calling out.

To help you cope:

- You might feel guilty about not answering every call, but remember that you have a life to lead. This is especially true at work and at night.

o o o

Paces, Shows Signs of Restlessness

You can tell where Kara's mother, Katrina, likes to walk. The carpet is noticeably dirtier in a distinct path from her bedroom, down the hall to the den, around the perimeter of the den, and back to her bedroom. Around 3 o'clock every afternoon, Katrina rises from the sofa and begins to walk this pattern as intently as if she were prayer-walking in a labyrinth.

"She does it for an hour or longer. I guess until she's tired," says Kara. "She used to welcome my kids, her grandkids, home from school, and they'd have a snack in the den. I wonder if that's what she's thinking about. But if you ask her, she ignores you. It's as if she isn't even aware of what she's doing."

WHY it happens:

Pacing—walking aimlessly or in a particular pattern around the home—is a common repetitive behavior or perseveration (the term for this behavior). Other examples include rocking, making repeated phone calls, picking at skin, and rummaging.

Pacing is typically caused by:

- *Anxiety or another form of distress.* What's bothering the person may be recent (a new caregiver, noise) or some long unresolved issue from the past.

- *Boredom,* feeling unproductive. Someone once used to a busy life may pace.

- *A need to use the bathroom* but an inability to say so.

- *A habitual impulse to move.* Former exercise-walkers, runners, or swimmers, for example, may pace if they can no longer walk outside for safety or stamina reasons.

- *A cognitive glitch.* The person "gets stuck" on a particular behavior pattern.

TRY this:

- **First address possible immediate needs**: Lead the person to the toilet and see if she needs to use it, for example.

- **Reinforce comforting routines**. Be sure to include some physical activity every day.

- **Ignore pacing that seems to calm rather than agitate**. At the same time, if it bothers you, look for alternate activities to counter possible boredom.

- **Make the house safer for walking**. If you haven't already done so, remove throw rugs, arrange furniture to make clear pathways, and get rid of clutter and low-to-the-ground hazards such as magazine racks, plants, extension cords, and pet toys.

- **Install night lighting**. Illuminate preferred safe paths—especially the hallways and rooms most used—with motion-sensitive nightlights, for example.

o o o

Picks at Skin, Clothes, or Small Objects

Ryan began to feel embarrassed about taking his father out in public. The older man's arms were dotted with red sores and half-healed scabs. He'd developed the habit of scratching at a dry spot on his skin while watching TV in the evening. Then when blood appeared, he'd pick at the edges. After a scab began to form, he'd pick at that, too, so old sores never completely healed even as he continued creating new ones.

When Ryan applied bandages, his dad picked those off, too.

WHY it happens:

Picking can refer to obsessively handling any number of different things: skin, labels, lint, pilling on sweaters, sticks, peeling paint. Some people pick at their hair or scalp.

The person might feel anxious about something in his or her current life, or something deep in the past, and the repetitive activity is soothing. He may not seem aware of the habit. For some chronic pickers, the compulsion is a way of gaining a sense of control in a life where they may feel little control (not unlike teenagers who cut themselves or those with an eating disorder, like bulimia).

Often, scratching the skin is triggered because of an irritant or a skin condition that makes skin dry and uncomfortable. Older skin can already be dry and fragile. Becoming dehydrated can also affect skin. In those situations, it's not unusual for someone with Alzheimer's to scratch or pick until skin bleeds.

TRY this:

- **Mention skin-picking to the doctor**. A professional can rule out or treat dry skin caused by a medication or other reversible cause.

- **Check the environment, if it's a new behavior**. Consider whether a new bath product, laundry detergent or dryer sheet, or medication might be irritating skin. Bed bugs, lice, or mosquito bites can also cause itching.

- **Be sure the hands are cleaned often to prevent infection, and keep nails trimmed short**. Apply a topical antibiotic such as Neosporin to open sores and try to cover with a bandage. Re-check often, as it also might get picked off.

- **Apply lots of moisturizer designed for dry skin to keep skin softer, especially after bathing**. Be sure the person drinks enough to ward off dehydration's drying effects.

- **Offer long-sleeve shirts to cover skin**. Lightweight cotton is most comfortable. Or try a wool, cashmere, or synthetic sweater that pills, as a satisfying but safer substitute to pick at than skin. Someone who picks at the scalp may consent to wearing a hat and lose the habit if his hands are diverted to something else.

- **Offer alternatives that keep the hands busy**. Examples: fidget spinners, finger puppets, worry beads, rubber de-stressing balls, a rubber-band ball, yarn to wind or a simple crocheting project, a toolbox to organize, clothes or towels to fold, lotion or nail polish to apply, a gadget to use (like an iPod), a junk drawer to organize.

- **For someone with more advanced-stage disease, consider an activity apron or lap pillow**. Both are designed for tactile stimulation, with different textures and things to handle sewn right on the fabric. Try searching online for "Alzheimer's activity apron."

- **Reinforce a sense of meaning and purpose**. Find ways to involve the person in household activities and express your gratitude often.

o o o

Rummaging

"What are you looking for, Ma?" asks Kate.

"Oh, I'll find it soon," Kate's mother, Dorothy, says evasively as she goes on opening and closing drawers, riffling through papers, old makeup, pencils, balls of string, and a jumble of other unrelated objects. The rummaging tends to start in the evening and can go on for an hour or more. Eventually, Dorothy picks out something—an old sock, masking tape, a turkey baster—and announces, "Ah, just what I was looking for!"

Some nights, though, she never "finds" the thing she thinks she needs.

WHY it happens:

Rummaging—restlessly and repeatedly going through drawers, papers, toolboxes, or similar collections of materials—is one of many repetitive behaviors some people with dementia show.

It can have several different (sometimes overlapping) causes:

- *Agitation or anxiety.* Moving the hands around is a way to channel a lack of ease.

- *Boredom.* It's simply something to do.

- *Lack of exercise.* Not moving around enough can come out as restless behaviors.

- *Feeling vulnerable, upset, or otherwise nervous.* As with other continuous behaviors, rummaging can be calming.

- *Chronic hoarding.* Someone who's a hoarder may be searching for a "saved" object.

TRY this:

- **Look for a trigger**. Does the behavior begin or increase when the person is tired or in the company of new people? Is there too much background noise? Could it be related to being left alone or not having anything to do?

- **Try not to dwell on the behavior**. Avoid saying, "Don't do that!" or "What on earth are you looking for?" Instead focus on the person's mood and the circumstances of her day.

- **Ask if she's looking for something**. It's possible that she has an item in mind but has forgotten where it is (or even what the object is, she just remembers she's searching). You don't need to go along with it to the point where you're rummaging, too. But a kind, normal response can be reassuring.

- **Suggest the person look in her favorite "go to" hiding places**. Common sites include a hamper or laundry bag, special drawers, freezers, or unusual spots, like sugar bowls and kitchen canisters, often things that have lids or open.

- **When in doubt, take the behavior as a possible sign of a need for comfort and reassurance**. Offer a hug.

- **Accept rummaging that isn't disruptive as a curious function of the disease and let the person have at it**. Just be sure to remove anything dangerous that could be handled and misused, such as sharp knives or guns. Redirect problematic rummaging (such as messing up critical work papers or rummaging in garbage) to a better alternative.

- **Create a dedicated box or junk drawer of similar materials**. Or introduce something else the person may enjoy handling. Things that have worked for other caregivers include coins, buttons, office miscellany, papers or junk mail, kitchen utensils, tools, and mixed beans to sort. If the person is prone to putting the objects in her mouth, choose accordingly for safety.

- **Find other ways to channel nervous energy that involve the hands**: balling yarn, working with hand tools, playing with worry beads or knotted string, filling envelopes, peeling potatoes or carrots, applying stamps to envelopes.

See also in this chapter: "Hoarding, Hiding, and Clutter"

o o o

Sundowning (Worsening Behaviors in Evening)

Len has come to dread dinnertime. He likes to eat well enough. It's what starts happening as he prepares the meal, and what comes after, that's getting harder to take. His wife, Doris, starts saying the craziest things.

"Watch out for the creepies!" she often says to herself or to him (he isn't sure which). "The creepies are coming! I know it, I know it!" She can't articulate who, or what, "creepies" are. She doesn't talk about them during the day. If he asks, she looks at him like he's crazy.

He used to turn on the TV so she could watch while he cooked, but she began to see the creepies in news programs and laundry commercials. Now he has her sit in the kitchen with him, but she can't sit still. She peeks out the windows and peers into cupboards. By day, Len can have a back-and-forth conversation with Doris. But not at dinnertime or after. For the rest of the evening, until she finally falls asleep exhausted, well past 10 (and well past when Len is worn out), she'll be wringing her hands and talking nonsense.

WHY it happens:

Also called "sundown syndrome" or "sundowner's," it's the name for an onset of increased agitation, confusion, and/or aggression that tends to strike in the late afternoon or evening, after the sun goes down. Someone with dementia who sundowns may pace, wander, lash out, yell, show mood swings, hallucinate, show increased paranoia, or become unusually resistant. (These behaviors can also happen separately from sundowning at any time of day. Or they may happen in more intensity as the day winds down.)

Researchers aren't entirely sure what triggers sundown syndrome but think it's related to a disruption of the internal body clock. All our bodies follow circadian rhythms, which govern when we sleep and waken, our activity, and the hormonal reactions that help our bodies run properly. For unknown reasons, people with dementia have a disturbed body clock. There's some research to show that aging eyes (even in people without dementia) take in less sunlight, which may affect circadian rhythms.

Researchers point to these possible causes or triggers for sundowning:

- A drop in blood pressure

- Hunger or a change in glucose levels

- Reduced sleep needs (or, conversely, being overtired)

- Pain

- Poor hearing or vision, which alters perception

- Depression

Several of these factors are probably connected, researchers think. For example, someone with dementia and macular degeneration (an eye condition) may become more confused and upset by evening shadows, especially if tired.

Sundowning happens more often in fall and winter (when there's less daylight) and as dementia progresses.

TRY this:

- **Try to identify patterns other than time of day**. Does the setting sun hit mirrors or windows in a bothersome way, for example? Does the house get noisier at dinnertime as family members come home?

- **If you can identify a trigger, work to eliminate it**. Take the person with dementia to a quiet room when the kids come home, for example. Trim back bushes or branches that create eerie shadows. See if lighting or mirrors cast upsetting movements in his or her line of vision.

- **Expose the person with dementia to ample sunlight, especially early in the day**. Make sure he or she gets strong morning sun, either by going outside or sitting near a window with the curtains open. On cloudy days, try placing a full-spectrum fluorescent lamp (2,500 to 5,000 lux) a few feet away for two or three hours in the morning while, say, watching TV.

- **Encourage movement**. Gentle exercise or an outing in the morning or midday may help her feel more tired at the end of the day, especially if you curb long naps.

- **Try not to let the person fall into a sleep-wake schedule that's wildly out-of-synch with yours**. Waken her relatively early in the day, even if it would be more convenient to let her sleep. Minimize all-afternoon napping.

- **Reinforce routines**. If things happen at a different time every day, the sundowning might worsen.

- **If dinner will be served late, make sure to offer a sustaining snack**. Ideally make it a complex carbohydrate or protein, like 100 percent whole-wheat toast with peanut butter or some low-fat string cheese.

- **As evening nears, increase soothing sleep cues**. Play soft music instead of TV (news shows and reality shows can be especially jarring). Serve warm milk or cocoa, or ice cream. Draw the shades and turn off some indoor lighting. Offer a hand massage while you have a quiet talk or listen to music.

- **Secure the exits**. Motion sensors, chimes, locks, or gates can prevent nighttime wandering out of the house.

- **Make sure eyeglasses and hearing aids are clean and functioning**. Someone with dementia will probably neglect to do this. Keep prescriptions current. An eye exam could reveal an undiagnosed problem, such as macular degeneration, for example.

- **If aggression or other behaviors become hard to handle, mention sundowning to the doctor**. Mood stabilizers or the hormone melatonin may be effective. Beware of over-the-counter sleep aids, however; these can interact badly with Alzheimer's medications. Best: Take all medications to the doctor so that they can be reviewed individually and together.

Tip: "I loaded the app GreyMatters on a tablet. I could personalize it with Dad's pictures and music, and we could either use it together or he'd sit there by himself once I got it started. It soothed him in the evening like nothing else." —R.R.

To help you cope:

- **Reassure yourself that you're not crazy (or faint of heart) if sundowning becomes a big problem for you**. Depending on how it plays out in a given person, it can be extremely taxing to deal with and disrupt the sleep of the entire household. In extreme cases, it can be the "straw that breaks the camel's back," making home care impossible. Try as many behavioral interventions as you can, then consider medication. At the very least, persistent disruptive sundowning is a red flag to get more help or begin to consider what you'll do when you can no longer provide care at home.

o o o

Trouble Using Familiar Gadgets

My Dad was a veritable Mr. Gadget. A mechanical engineer and a gifted car mechanic, he was a natural and enthusiastic early adopter of color TVs, portable TVs, pocket calculators, CD players, car phones, cell phones, and camcorders. Into his 80s, he embraced desktop computers, digital cameras, home photo printers, and iPods.

It was especially distressing, then, to watch him at the bank one day deep into his dementia: He repeatedly jammed the wrong plastic card into an ATM. Finally, with help, he inserted the correct bank card only to be baffled by the buttons and options that followed.

Another time, a stopped clock drove him crazy. He checked his watch often and knew its time was wrong. And his instinct to tinker and repair remained strong. So he kept taking the clock off the wall to "fix" it. But by the time he pried off the back cover and inspected it, he could go no farther. He'd grunt and touch the control knob but utterly lacked the wherewithal to actually replace the batteries, re-set the time, replace the back, and return the clock to the wall. Over and over, I'd find the abandoned repair job, put it back together, and replace it on the wall. (In retrospect...I know! Why didn't I just get it repaired or hide it from view?!)

The telephone was an ongoing source of stress. When it rang and my mom would motion for him to pick up an extension, he'd choose one of several different TV and stereo remotes and start talking into it. (They were all black and full of buttons.) —P.S.S.

WHY it happens:

Understanding the use of many common objects recedes as Alzheimer's progresses. That can include the mastery of gadgetry we take for granted—phones, laptops, microwaves. In part it's because these are relatively complex tools that require an ability to follow a sequence of steps to use and a memory of the details involved, such as what a particular button represents. Newer gadgets like a coffee machine with capsules or home-automation tools (like Amazon Echo) may be misunderstood first because a longtime habit was never established in the first place.

Eventually someone with dementia stops recognizing objects for what they are. Even a simple tool like a toothbrush can confound.

TRY this:

- **Be patient if you get a new version of an old device**. (Common examples include a new TV remote with different buttons, an upgraded phone, or a microwave that's configured differently from the old one.) Learning new things is very difficult by mild stage dementia. Even someone who managed the old device well may find it difficult to learn how to use one that's slightly different.

- **Try using memory aids**. Circle the "on" button with permanent marker. Leave a note boiled down to two simple instructions ("Press red button. Then press yellow one."). Over time, however, even these may be hard to follow.

- **Avoid storing similar gadgets near each other**. A cell phone and a camera, or a house phone and a TV remote, for example, are often confused for each other.

- **Look for simplified versions of devices**. There are laptops that only do e-mail, "memory" phones whose buttons have pictures of the people most often dialed, and dial-less telephones that can be answered but not dialed. Learning to use even simple new devices can be challenging, however, and they're only short-term solutions as skills and cognition will decline.

- **Try not to criticize mistakes**. Just gently offer your help: "Let me see if I can do it."

- **Simplify the household**. Phase out gadgets that create consternation and confusion.

Tip: **"To give my mom something to look at without her having to change channels, I put on long, two- to three-hour DVDs. Sometimes nature shows, sometimes cartoons. No commercials and no buttons to push." — J.M.L.**

o o o

Undresses in Public

"I'm hot," Mildred announced to her family, gathered for her birthday. Ten minutes later, she reappeared in the dining room. She'd changed from her heavy sweater into a light blouse—and nothing else. No pants, no panties.

Her daughter Marie shrieked. Her grandchildren started snickering. "What's the matter? Haven't you ever felt like being free?" Mildred said, waggling her wrinkled hips.

Says Marie: "Not a week later, Mom said she was hot at a restaurant and started to undo the snaps on her blouse, right at the table. She got the whole thing off almost before any of us realized it. When the poor waiter, a teenage boy, stared, she said, 'Haven't you ever seen a bra before, honey?'"

WHY it happens:

The checks-and-balances in the brain that prevent us from doing or saying whatever we feel like in the moment can erode as part of dementia's brain changes. A person may gradually lose the ability to recognize what's socially appropriate behavior along with the ability to stop herself. This loss of inhibition is known as disinhibition.

Someone may start to disrobe because he or she:

- Feels too hot

- Is uncomfortable (itchy tag, bra too snug, scratchy fabric, etc.)

- Needs to use the bathroom

- Is having a delusion and therefore not fully aware of the actual context

- Is sexually aroused

- Is bored

TRY this:

- **Look first for the quick fix**. See if you can connect the behavior to a specific cause you can remedy, such as scratchy fabrics or the temperature in the room.

- **Be low-key and matter-of-fact**: "No, we don't do that here. Let me help you find a shirt that's cooler (or that you like better)." If you're in public or with others, cover the person and calmly and quietly escort her to a more private place. Some caregivers travel with a shawl for handy coverage in a pinch.

- **Look for soft, seamless undergarments, sweatpants, and tops**. Know that clothing can irritate older, dry skin, so the person wants to shed it. All-cotton is usually more comfortable than synthetic. Cashmere and fleece are softer and less itchy than wool.

- **If undressing becoming a chronic problem, make it harder to do**. Try introducing coveralls, jumpsuits, or shirts without buttons or that button in the back. Some makers offer special clothes that are designed to be hard to get out of. Search online for "Alzheimer's clothing." Beware, though, that these choices can be counterproductive if the person needs to use the bathroom often. Another catch is that you'll have to help with the dressing more than you may already do now.

- **Use redirection to provide something else to do**. You may be able to persuade someone beyond mild-stage dementia for whom this is an ongoing issue to wear a "busy apron" onto which zippers, buttons, ribbons, dangling keys, and other hand-occupying things have been sewn.

- **Ask the doctor to review medications that may be contributing to dry skin**. In some cases, the solution may be as simple as treating this issue.

To help you cope:

- **Let go of worries about propriety and what others might think**. The person isn't trying to embarrass you or mortify you. When you remember it's just the disease at work, it's easier to find the calm you'll need to handle it.

o o o

Upset by Reflection in Mirror

Lately Jack had become reluctant to take a shower. "I don't like being watched," he complained. His wife, Ann, assured him that she wasn't watching. She would just be waiting outside the door like always, with a warm towel and fresh pajamas. "I'm being stalked. I know it," he insisted.

One day as Jack and Ann walked down the hall, he grabbed her arm and froze. "Don't move! There he is again! Call the police!" Ann panicked and tried to follow his gaze. A framed mirror hung in an alcove at the end of the hall. Her heart sank. The "intruder" Jack saw—as well as, she now realized, the "bathroom stalker"— was her husband's own reflection.

WHY it happens:

Just as someone loses the ability to recognize longtime acquaintances, he can lose the ability to register his own reflection as himself. A moving image in a mirror can seem like a separate person, either vaguely familiar or a stranger.

Some people with dementia befriend this "person." They have pleasant conversations with their reflection. If it's a source of entertainment and pleasure and doesn't cause someone to grow agitated or upset, there's no reason to discourage the behavior.

One caregiver reported finding her mother washing the face of her own reflection!

TRY this:

- **Remove or cover any mirrors that become bothersome**. Or cover them with a large towel, cloth, or curtain.

- **If a medicine cabinet has a mirrored door, try replacing it with a solid door**. Or remove the door and leave the open shelving. Remove any dangerous substances, such as medications or mouthwash that the person with dementia might swallow accidentally.

- **If it's a large wall-sized mirror** (as in many modern bathrooms): Try hanging a curtain or shower curtain rod over the top, so the curtain can be open or closed. It may seem very odd to you or your guests, but to your loved one, the mirror may come to be "out of sight, out of mind."

- **Switch to using hand mirrors or portable makeup mirrors for yourself.** Store a full-length mirror inside a closet, where it can't be accidentally glimpsed.

- **Look to see if reflective glass on a painting or framed poster is having the same effect.** You might need to relocate the piece.

- **Consider if hallucinations are part of the problem.** It may not be solely a reflection issue if the person with dementia continues to talk about people "watching" or "intruders."

(See also in this chapter: "Hallucinates: Sees and Hears Things That Aren't There.")

o o o

Wanders Off

A senior center in Germany had a growing problem: Its residents occasionally would decide they wanted to go "home" or visit relatives and would walk away to look for the nearest bus to take them home.

Solution: Staffers installed a replica of the town's familiar green and yellow bus signs right outside the door, next to a bench. Their long-term memory intact, residents would recognize the distinctive sign and sit down at the "bus stop" to wait. That delayed the wanderers long enough for staffers to find them.

"The bus is delayed," they'd explain. "Would you like to come in for a cup of coffee while you wait?" The residents would come back inside and promptly forget about their earlier decision to leave.

These phantom bus stops have since popped up in other care homes in the country.

WHY it happens:

At root, people wander because of cognitive changes that cause confusion, disorientation, and other inabilities to recognize what they're doing, where they are, or how to get back.

If the person in your care hasn't wandered off yet, prepare yourself as if he or she will. About three out of every five people with Alzheimer's wander at some point—that is, they'll leave home of their own free will but become too confused or lost to make it back home on their own. Usually they're going about normal activities (like taking a walk, going to get the mail, intending to run an errand). It's not that they sneak off or run away.

And if someone disappears once, he's more likely to do so again. Some experts say it can take six to eight episodes before family members recognize a pattern or the danger the behavior poses.

The label "wandering" sounds a lot more pleasant than the experience: Every year older adults with Alzheimer's are found nearly frozen or dehydrated, hit by cars, mugged, or even drowned or otherwise dead after having wandered off. Of those who are not located within 24 hours, half will be seriously or fatally injured, according to the Alzheimer's Association.

Wandering is especially dangerous because people with dementia don't usually think they're lost. So they don't ask for help or directions. They often don't even respond to their own name as searchers call. Some hide instinctively. Others insist, when found, that they're not lost at all, confounding searchers. Police say that 90 percent of wanderers are found within a five-mile radius of where they disappeared.

Someone with dementia may take off due to...

- *Habit.* Someone used to walking, jogging, or driving may take off to do so, only to falter midway—unsure of the location or how to get back. People often leave for "work" at a certain time of day. The sight of a coat on a peg may trigger the habit of putting it on and walking out the door.

- *Fear or anxiety.* Too much noise (at a party, for example) or a perceived threat may trigger flight.

- *A sensation of loss.* Someone feeling upset about missing something (literally or figuratively) may wander off to seek it.

- *Curiosity.* People with Alzheimer's live in the moment. A passing truck, bird, or other distraction can pique interest and the person follows it along. Someone in a new residence may wander off to explore.

TRY this:

To prevent wandering:

- **Know the warning signs**. People are candidates for wandering and getting lost if they begin to return from normal outings (like walks or drives) later than usual or if they try to "go home" when at home already or to "go to work" when they're retired. Be wary if the person seems bored or restless or gets upset in a public space. Not being able to find a public restroom or other common location is another red flag.

If the person has been late or gone missing at least once:

Consider possible triggers:

- **Have there been any big changes in the person's life?** A recent move or a new caregiver, for example, can be stressful. In demanding times, reinforce a comforting routine. Consider making fewer outings.

- **Have any medications changed?** Agitation could be a side effect. Mention the wandering to the prescribing doctor.

- **Is there a pattern to the wandering episodes?** If it always happens at night, for example, it could indicate fear or loneliness—he may need extra support after dark. If it's at mealtimes, he may be hungry or thirsty and unable to follow through on these desires. Some people wander at specific times linked to activities from their work life or other former routines. Target those times with new, engrossing activities that distract from the impulse to take off.

- **Is the wanderer busy enough?** Ideally, aim for a daily schedule that includes a variety of different activities, outdoor time if possible, and social time. Having a routine and a full, diverse schedule are two of the best ways to minimize wandering. Being busy by day also makes it more likely he'll sleep through the night.

Create a safe wandering environment, if you can. While this isn't an option for every family, if you have a yard that can be secured, you might be able to enhance it for controlled wandering. Set the yard with winding paths or a labyrinth to pace, for example.

Reduce temptations to wander. Some ideas:

- **Keep keys out of sight**. Someone who has Alzheimer's that's severe enough to include wandering shouldn't be driving. But he may still recognize keys left hanging in a familiar place and drive off—even if you think he has no longer remembers how to drive.

- **Make doors to the outside hard to open**. Try plastic grip-style doorknob covers found in childproofing catalogs or sites. These can be too difficult for an older person with dementia to open. Jam sliding doors with a strip of wood in the bottom of the frame.

- **Consider changing locks**. Any kind of door lock that's different from what the person has always used might work because it's hard for someone with cognitive impairment to learn new things. Try a chain lock in a higher-than usual position or a key lock for a door than once had a button lock.

- **Disguise dangerous doorways**. A gentle alternative to door locks is to lead the person away from certain doors with visual cues that convey that the door is something else. Camouflage possibilities include painting the door to match a surrounding wall or hanging a mirror or a poster of scenery (which might be perceived as a window). You can also buy or paint a mural on the door designed to make it look like a bookshelf or pantry shelf. Some families have had success hanging a "Do not enter" or "STOP" sign on an exit door.

- **Position a solid black mat in front of doorways**. To some people with cognitive impairment, the black square reads like a hole, making them afraid to cross the threshold.

- **Skip the lectures and logic**. Telling someone with dementia, "Don't do that again" will be as effective as telling a toddler not to run off. Neither has the cognitive capacity to remember the conversation or act on it. Remember that someone who wanders once is likely to wander again.

More safety strategies:

- **Avoid crowds**. Crowded situations—shopping malls, big parties, outdoor plazas and events—can produce stress that leads to wandering off not just in that place but even once you're back home. It's also harder for you to keep track of each other in a crowd; you can't be distracted for a moment.

- **Avoid leaving a wanderer in the car alone**. While you're running a quick errand in the bank or drugstore, he's liable to become frightened or worried (five minutes can feel like an hour) and slip out of the vehicle.

- **Look into alarms that signal movement**. These include bed pads or chair pads with wireless remote alarms that offer an immediate alert when someone gets up. Look for them online. Other devices include floor mats with remote alarms, motion detectors that send alerts directly to a caregiver, and conventional door chimes that sound when a door is opened. Or go low tech: One caregiver hung Christmas bells in such a way that they jingled loudly whenever the door opened.

- **Tell immediate neighbors about your loved one's Alzheimer's and tendency to wander**. Ask them to call you if he uncharacteristically comes over to visit or is seen walking alone.

- **Look into adult day programs or a relief caregiver when you must go out**. You can't leave a wanderer home alone safely even for short periods.

- **Avoid using restraints**. Aside from being inhumane, they've been shown to cause injury. Locking someone in his room can cause anxiety and aggression that persists for days -- and only make him more prone to wander.

- **Keep hallways and walking paths inside the living area clear and easy to meander in**. Some people are satisfied wandering indoors.

Tip: **"I started to take Dad to the gym with me. He couldn't do much, but he liked it and the extra activity seemed to wear him out. He slept better and stopped trying to leave the house." —M.C.**

Prepare in advance for not being able to locate your loved one:

- **Enroll in a search program**. MedicAlert + Alzheimer's Association Safe Return is a 24-hour nationwide emergency-response system for people with Alzheimer's or other forms of dementia. Along with calling 911, you can call an 800-number to activate a search that involves local Alzheimer's Association chapters and local law enforcement. Identification jewelry is provided as part of this fee-based service. Also ask if your local police station, sheriff, fire department, or other emergency responder participates in Project Lifesaver, a public-safety program that uses tracking technology to find lost wanderers. Costs vary by area, and it requires the person to wear a small tracking device.

  Note: It's really smart to enroll someone with dementia in a program now, even if there's never been a wandering incident. After *Washington Post* writer Tom Jackman's father went missing, he discovered there was a 10-month wait to get in his local Project Lifesaver. Jackman's dad, 78, drove from his home in Virginia to Baltimore, until he ran out of gas. Luckily he was found safe, 20 hours later, though he couldn't recall why he'd gone there—a first-time incident.

- **Use identification**. Safe return-type programs often provide identification to wear. It's also a good idea to write the name, disease, and your phone number inside the jacket the person wears, as well as on a piece of paper in his wallet.

- **Pay attention to your loved one's wardrobe**. It's helpful to searchers if you can identify what the person was wearing when he or she went missing. One idea: Pare down a chronic wanderer's wardrobe to multiples that look the same.

- **Keep a recent photo handy**. Many families avoid photographing a loved one with Alzheimer's because the disease and age can seem to alter his or her familiar appearance. But an up-to-date portrait will help searchers tremendously.

- **Take advantage of GPS technology**. Cellphones can be programmed to activate GPS, but many people with Alzheimer's no longer carry phones (or never did), or have outdated models. One option is to wear a phone on a belt or a pair of "smart" shoes containing GPS sensors. (Search online for "Alzheimer's GPS shoe.")

Tip: **"I got rid of Dad's dark shirts but kept the brightest Aloha-prints he liked, along with his solid orange and yellow polos. That way he was easier to spot when he wandered off." —E.R.**

If someone does go missing...

- **Call 911; don't hesitate**. Don't wait for the usual "missing for 24 hours" rule of thumb to take effect. Especially in very hot or cold weather, it's best to call for help within 15 minutes. With impaired judgment and memory loss, someone with Alzheimer's who's lost is in harm's way and needs help getting home. In addition to local systems for locating missing older adults with dementia, the majority of states have Silver Alert systems (public notifications about missing, impaired older adults) that authorities can activate.

- **Know where to look**. Most who walk (not drive) off are found within a mile of home. In a University of Florida analysis of 675 incidents involving the Alzheimer's Association Safe Return program, one in four wanderers turned up in a residential yard. About one in five were found standing in streets. Others turned up at senior centers, restaurants, shopping centers, and other businesses.

Other studies have shown that wanderers often are found in ditches and creeks and behind bushes and briars, usually not far from a road. Two-thirds cross a road at some point.

To help you cope:

- **Try not to take wandering as a criticism of you or your care**. It's rarely an attempt to "escape" a disliked situation. That would involve more premeditation and planning than most people with Alzheimer's are capable of. The relatives of good, loving, and attentive caregivers still wander.

o o o

SEXUALITY-RELATED CHALLENGES

Makes Inappropriate Advances

*"Shari, baby! Where've you been? Your knockers are calling me!"
the man said, wiggling his fingers as he reached toward his
attractive visitor's breasts.*

*"Dad! I'm not Sharon, um, Mom. I'm Sue, your daughter," she
replied, jumping back.*

*Her father looked confused for a second. "Well then how about a
kiss?"*

*Sue approached her father for a hug, quickly turning her cheek in
case he gave her the wrong kind of kiss.*

WHY it happens:

Many people with dementia still have sexual urges—and want to act
on them. But with poor impulse control and self-censorship, and
lacking the ability to read a social situation as they once did, these
feelings can lead someone to behave in inappropriate ways.

Advances can range from suggestive comments to propositioning,
and from flirtatious touches to groping. Anyone can be a target for
the advances: a caregiver, a daughter, an old friend, a virtual
stranger. The advances seldom reveal some long-simmering desire
now being acted on (as caregivers often believe). Your husband with
Alzheimer's making a pass at your best friend of 30 years isn't proof
of his secret crush or their past affair, for example, and shouldn't be
taken that way. The target is usually someone who's handy out of
sheer proximity.

Sometimes a parent mistakes an adult child for his or her spouse,
leading to awkward moments. The person with dementia isn't
thinking incest, of course; he really believes the adult child is
someone else. Bathing is a common trigger. Sexual
inappropriateness can also be a bid for attention.

Disinhibition (lack of self-control) about sex is thought to affect up
to one in four people with dementia. Men and women are about
equally affected, according to a 2005 article in the British journal
Advances in Psychiatric Treatment, although sexual complaints
about men are more common. For unknown reasons (possibly
better reporting but also the sheer number of people living
together), it's more often seen in nursing homes. This behavior can

increase as the disease progresses before finally subsiding in late-stage Alzheimer's.

Things that can contribute include a lack of a regular partner (such as in a widower who develops dementia), boredom, or misinterpreting cues seen on TV or overheard. People who struggled to contain hypersexual behavior when they were healthy often behave inappropriately now. Delirium, a behavior syndrome caused by a physical stress such as an infection or pain, can also cause sexually inappropriate behavior.

TRY this:

- **If the behavior is sudden and new**: Consider a medical evaluation to rule out delirium.

- **If the behavior is ongoing, see if you can identify and remove a trigger for the behavior**. Is it always directed to a particular person? (If it's an aide, for example, you might need to make a staff change.) Does it happen on days the routine is disrupted? When the person drinks? During help with personal care?

- **Make sure the person isn't drinking too much**. Alcohol can add to disinhibition in someone with dementia just as in someone with a healthy brain.

- **Try not to shame the person with dementia or make him feel embarrassed**. Act as neutrally as you can muster. At the same time, gently but firmly set a boundary. "That's not how we say hello." "Please don't talk that way, okay?" "You can't put your hand there." "I can't help you if you do that."

- **Restate your relationship**: "Hi, Dad, it's your middle daughter, Sue!" "Look: Mrs. Smith, the hairdresser, has come to trim your hair."

Tip: **"My sister-in-law used humor with my dad (her father-in-law): 'You old devil! You know I'm a married woman, so you'd better stop, or Jack might beat you up!'"** —K. S.

- **Know it's also okay not to take it**. If you feel threatened, walk away or leave the room if you can.

- **Quickly use distraction to get the person's mind off sexual activity**. Find a fresh activity or move to a different room. Offering a snack can satisfy a different kind of physical craving.

- **Avoid friendly flirtatiousness or sexual-type teasing**, which might be misinterpreted. At the same time, some people will act less sexually if they have increased platonic physical affection—hand holding, hugs, even walking arm in arm or dancing together. You have to see what works in your specific case.

- **If helping with bathing is a trigger, have someone of the same sex handle this task**. You may need to hire a home aide just for this, or enlist a relative.

- **Strange but true creative solutions**: A 68-year-old man with dementia in one facility turned his advances to a three-foot-tall Pink Panther doll and stopped trying to molest staff, according to a report in the *American Journal of Geriatric Psychiatry*. The long, soft proportions of a body pillow might also comfort someone accustomed to having a bed partner.

- **If the problem is severe, mention it to a doctor**. Meds that can be used to treat sexual disinhibition include antiandrogens (hormone treatment that impairs sexual functioning), mood stabilizers, antidepressants, and antipsychotics (a last-resort drug for people with dementia because they can cause other problems).

To help you cope:

- **Know that for an adult child, this can be one of the more distressing problems to deal with**. It's even harder when you or your child is the target of the unwanted advances. The mix of shock, distaste, guilt, and confusion you may feel is absolutely normal. It's the ultimate muddling of your social roles.

- **Some caregivers find talking to a counselor or therapist helpful**. That's not because they've done anything amiss but to gain perspective and coping advice.

- **Remind friends and visitors who are targeted that the disease is causing this behavior**. Some caregivers report losing "shocked" friends over this, but more typical is for people to be deeply empathetic. If a friend grows reluctant to visit in person, try to schedule visits when the person is asleep or when there's back-up help, as it's also important for you to have time with friends.

o o o

Makes Unwanted Advances to Spouse

Cora has begun to dread evening, especially bedtime. She and Stanislaus, her husband of 57 years, have a good marriage, and she still loves him. But his sex drive is still strong, and increasingly, this troubles her.

"In the first few years after he was diagnosed, when we were intimate was like being with the old Stan. He seemed fine," she says. "But as he's become more child-like and needs more help from me, I just don't like thinking of him that way [sexually] any more. It makes me uncomfortable."

WHY it happens:

We're sexual beings. The instincts and habits that make up our sexuality are deeply rooted. People with mild- and moderate-stage dementia continue to become aroused and have desire. Many couples find intimacy to be a source of mutual comfort and reassurance at a turbulent time. Your loved one may even seem more like his or her "old self" during sex.

For many couples, though, the desire to have sex can dissipate early in the disease process, especially on the side of the caregiving spouse, and these feelings of disconnection grow as the disease progresses. The partner's increasing dependency changes the way they view their intimate relationship and makes desire wane. Stress and exhaustion take a toll, too. Some mates say they feel like they're "giving" something to a confused partner who expresses desire, even though they themselves are no longer sexually attracted. More commonly, caregiving mates grow turned off by cognitive changes and wrestle with guilt or sexual frustration. Still other caregiving spouses believe sex under later-stage circumstances is unethical because their loved one is incapable of fully understanding what he's doing. (Indeed, some people with dementia become frightened or upset by advances made toward them.)

Should you? Shouldn't you? What's right? "There are a lot more questions than answers," says geriatric psychiatrist Ken Robbins. The "right" answer to what one's sex life looks like after a dementia diagnosis is completely personal.

TRY this:

In general:

- **Ask yourself what your partner would think if your positions were reversed**. Do you still feel sex is a marital "duty" if you aren't interested and your partner is impaired? What does your conscience tell you? It's an entirely individual call, but those kinds of questions can be a useful tool to help you think things through.

- **Consider talking to a therapist if you're conflicted, distressed, or sad**. A neutral third party can help you sort out your feelings.

In the moment:

- **If you're not comfortable having sex, make up a white lie**. Your partner may quickly forget when the urge passes.

- Substitute other nonsexual forms of giving physical affection, such as a shoulder rub or holding hands. It may be enough to satisfy the person's need for touch and reassurance.

- **Use distraction**. Change activities to something absorbing (a car ride, playing with a pet). Or offer a favorite snack: "Let's have a cookie first."

To help you cope:

- **Remind yourself that even when a sexual relationship falters, couples can still have intimacy**. Talking, touching, hand-holding, spending time together, and just knowing that you're there seeing your partner through his or her chronic illness can reinforce close feelings.

- **Consider separate sleeping arrangements**. You don't have to make a big deal about it, but let it evolve. One caregiving spouse stayed up later each night and would go to another room to sleep. Her husband, a sound sleeper, didn't notice, and she'd awaken first.

What About Sex Outside Your Marriage?

Support groups and others report rising numbers of Alzheimer's caregivers contemplating sexual relationships outside of marriage.

Given that Alzheimer's can be a long disease, and many partners are still in their prime sexual years themselves—especially in the rising numbers of early-onset cases—the math can be daunting. Obviously this is a decision with many personal considerations. Some believe the vow of "'til death do us part" means that the well partner should hang tough for the duration, period. Others believe that marriage vows are made between two parties of sound mind, and that pledges should be allowed to change when one of those minds becomes unsound.

This is one dilemma, caregivers consistently say, where those who haven't experienced Alzheimer's firsthand might hold their tongues before weighing in with an opinion. Companionship changes. Sharing changes. A relationship rocked by Alzheimer's is no longer equal or reciprocal. The loss of the sexual dimension of a long, happy partnership can layer more stress and sadness on the healthy spouse who's already grappling with so many losses. These are incalculably tough things to come to terms with. (And if the partnership wasn't happy, that adds another troubling factor in the mix.)

As Richard Anderson, past-president of the Well Spouse Association puts it, "The emotional well-being of both partners is paramount."

Ultimately it's a decision only you and your conscience can make.

What helps:

- **Talk to a trusted therapist or clergyperson**. (Know that clergy have come down on both sides of this ethical dilemma.) Beware of input from friends, who may have trouble separating their own personal agenda from your dilemma or may not be able to fully relate.

- **Realize that adult children have their own vested interests**. They may be grappling with denial about the Alzheimer's or not want to think too closely about their parents' intimate relationship. They may have some unrelated, unresolved issue with a parent that colors their view. In the end, your sex life isn't their business now any more than it ever was.

o o o

Masturbates Publicly

Mary Jo began to avoid bringing her kids to visit Grandpa Joel. One day, she left them all watching cartoons together in the family room while she made sandwiches in the kitchen with her mom. When she poked her head in the room to call them all to lunch, she saw Grandpa Joel sitting in his recliner with his hands in his pants.

"The kids didn't notice, but I was mortified," she says. "I don't know what set him off—something in the cartoon, or what. Maybe he does that all the time, but I was too embarrassed to even ask my mom about it."

WHY it happens:

As with making inappropriate advances, this kind of sexual behavior happens because people with dementia lose the ability to judge what's socially acceptable. They may act on impulse more and lack self-control (disinhibition).

Sometimes people with dementia who masturbate actually have to use the toilet. They may fumble with their clothes for that reason and then forget the need to urinate and fondle themselves instead.

Examples of related behaviors: undressing in public, purposely exposing one's self, and viewing pornography (magazines, videos) when others are present.

TRY this:

- **If the behavior is recent and new, have the person evaluated**. There may be delirium, a urinary tract infection, prostate trouble (in men), or another treatable physical cause.

- **See if you can identify a trigger**. Does a person, situation, or time of day seem to set off the behavior?

- **Avoid shaming**. It's counterproductive.

- **Escort the person to a private place**. If it's a bedroom or bathroom, say, "You can only do that in here."

- **Distract**. Offer a snack or something else to do.

- **Provide hands-on activities at times when the masturbation typically occurs**. Working with the hands can be an effective distraction and deterrent.

- **Look into clothing that's more difficult to remove**. Some caregivers report success dressing a man in overalls without a front fly.

- **If the problem is severe, mention it to a doctor**. Meds that may be used to treat sexual disinhibition include antiandrogens (hormone treatment that impairs sexual functioning), mood stabilizers, antidepressants, and antipsychotics (a last-resort drug for people with dementia because they can cause other problems).

o o o

PERSONAL CARE CHALLENGES

Dislikes Bathing or Showering, or Won't

"I'm not dirty! I'm not dirty!" Hal insists whenever his wife, Evelyn, asks if he wants to get in the shower first. She tries to ignore the fact that her once-fastidious husband hasn't bathed or showered in days. She playfully wipes any bits of food from his face after meals, and she makes sure his hair is cut regularly so it doesn't get oily and matted. But after a week or two, she can't ignore the body odor any more.

Sometimes, Hal surprises her by hopping under the running water when she asks. Other times, half the day goes by trying to cajole him into cleaning up.

WHY it happens:

Because bathing is a deeply held habit, the person may at first remember to do it. But gradually the sequence of steps may become too difficult to manage. Avoiding it altogether becomes easier.

Often other factors contribute to a refusal to bathe:

- *Discomfort.* Maybe the water is too cold or too hot. Maybe the air temperature varies too much. It's also stressful to stay balanced while trying to not slip.

- *Water!* It's common for people with dementia to dislike the feeling of water over the face and head.

- *Pain.* A frail person might find the whole business physically overwhelming.

- *Modesty.* Being helped by someone of the opposite gender— even a spouse—can make a bather feel self-conscious, shy, or deeply embarrassed.

- *Dignity.* Having to be helped bathing represents neediness and makes people feel juvenile or even disrespected, especially when help is provided in a brusque or insensitive way or invades personal space in an abrupt way.

- *Defensiveness.* The more you cajole, the more a reluctant bather may dig in. It's easier to do nothing. (It's no longer about the bath; now it's about a power struggle.)

- *Fear.* Fear of falling is common. One bad experience—a slip, a rough helper, being chilled—can understandably make someone wary of repeating the experience. The incident itself may be forgotten, but the sound of water running or the sight of the tub remains vaguely agitating.

TRY this:

To encourage bathing:

- **Start by reinforcing a routine**. Bathing should happen at the same time every day—ideally when and how he always did it, even if it's not the most convenient for you or a helper. (First thing in the morning? Before bed? Shower or bath?) The power of routine is such that it can be much easier to bathe someone every day rather just twice a week.

- **Just start preparations**. Avoid asking how long it's been since the last shower or if the person wants one ("no!"), or talking about how much it's needed.

- **Get as many things ready in advance as possible**. Heat up the room to a comfortable temperature. Have toiletries and towels ready. If you have to leave the person alone to retrieve something, he may give up and leave.

- **Try leading the person to a prepared bath**—as if you were walking somewhere else—without talking about it. The idea isn't to surprise but to minimize hesitation. Once there, mention the benefits: "You always like that clean, calm feeling after your bath. Then you'll be ready for ice cream."

- **Pay attention to your body language**. Remember, to get someone to do something, it helps to smile or sing, seem relaxed, and be encouraging.

Tip: **"I would tell Mom, 'Remember that smell Dad got when he'd get dirty? I think you're starting to have some of that. It's hard to smell on your own self, I know. Maybe today would be a nice day for a bath.'" —A.K.**

- **Go bit-by-bit**. Say, "How about we just get your feet wet?" Stress how relaxing it feels. Once the shoes and socks are off and the feet washed, try hands next. Then say you'd like to wash the arms, then the back. Cover what you've just cleaned with a dryer-warmed towel. Starting with one body part at a time can often coax someone through a complete sponge bath.

- **Give your loved one a washcloth to hold**, even if he isn't capable of doing the work. That keeps the hands busy and feels "right." Encourage someone who's able to clean to do as much as possible. Don't do it all for him.

- **Another way to coax someone who's reluctant:** spilling a little juice or sauce "by accident." "Oh, look what I did! Let me help you out of that...well, since you're changing, let's wash up, so you won't have to bother later."

To increase comfort:

- **Help the person associate bathing with positive feelings by making it as pleasant an experience as possible**. With time and patience, this can also help someone who's skittish because of a previous bad experience. Linking the activity to a reward (say, after-bath ice cream) also does this.

- **Employ distractions**. Set up a music player and play soft big band music or jazz. A sports fan might like to listen to a game on the radio. Consider a lava lamp, a portable TV, or fish bowl to look at if there's room and it's safe.

- **Try warming towels and robe in the dryer for 10 minutes before they're needed**. They'll retain warmth and feel cozy, adding to the positive associations with bathtime.

- **Install a bath bench**. They're available at medical supply stores, home stores, or online. Being seated can raise a sense of security in the shower or make sponge baths easier in the tub. Secure grab bars are also worth the small investment.

- **Use a hand-held shower nozzle**. It's easier to control the flow of water, and you can keep it away from the face and hair.

- **For someone struggling with modesty**, use small towels to cover genitals and breasts. Then wash underneath them.

- **Avoid bath oils**. These can make skin slippery and hard to hold, and make the floor slippery too.

- **Keep up a patter of conversation**. Talk about a TV show or news about relatives—anything that distracts from the personal nature of what you're doing.

- **Cover the mirror**. Around moderate-stage dementia, a reflection or movement noticed within it can be perceived as a stranger "watching." This can raise inhibition.

- **Options for washing hair**: Some bathers find a scalp massage during shampooing a delight, especially if you take care to keep water out of the face with a hand-nozzle and a washcloth to cover the eyes. Others prefer dry shampoo products. You can also wash hair using a washcloth by dabbing on a small amount of shampoo and rinsing it out with a clean wet cloth. Or leave hair washing for part of a weekly salon or barbershop appointment.

- **Find the right pace**. If you go too slowly, the person may get chilled. Go too fast, and he'll feel rushed and irritated.

To help you cope:

- **Reconsider frequency**. A daily ritual might be easier to get through than an irregular one. On the other hand, a daily bath probably isn't necessary if the habit has been lost. Try a daily "top and tail" (face and genitals) and a weekly bath.

- **Consider this task as a good excuse for enlisting outside help**. If the person is just too resistant or if you're having any kind of physical trouble (such as a bad back or struggling to help someone heavier than you), try hiring a home aide of the same gender as your loved one to come just once or twice a week for bathing. If professional help isn't in the cards, maybe there's a family member better suited to the task who can take it on—a son to help a father, say.

o o o

Dressing: Chooses Inappropriate Clothes

As her dementia progressed, my mother-in-law's favorite outfit seemed to be a navy tracksuit made of heavy fleece. It was nothing like the smart sweaters, trousers, and coordinating jewelry she'd always worn. But I could see the appeal: It was easy to put on and take off, and comfortable.

One hot summer day, arriving for a visit, we were knocked over by a wave of heat when opening the front door. The air-conditioning in her house was broken. It was 95 degrees. But Louie was wearing her usual fleece tracksuit. It had become her go-to uniform—winter or summer, air conditioning or no air conditioning. —P.S.S.

WHY it happens:

Loss of judgment and decision-making ability leave the person unable to weigh factors like weather, season, and occasion to make sensible choices. It can be complicated for any of us to figure out the appropriate thing to wear each day. For someone with dementia, this can lead to lots of mix-ups, like light jackets in blizzards, sequins at the local diner, or sporting gear at church.

Clothing involves many parts to coordinate and assemble, adding to the challenge. It's easy to get overwhelmed by the options.

TRY this:

- **Simplify the choices**. Pare down closets and drawers, so they contain a limited number of appropriate options.

- **Change out closets with the seasons**. Make sure the only choices that are accessible suit the season. Store bulky sweaters in boxes in another room during the summer, for example.

- **Lay out the next day's outfits**. Layer them in the order they're to be put on—so underclothes are on top, above shirts and pants.

- **Make sure all the clothes are easy-on, easy-off**. Most people have success with elastic waistbands, popover sweaters, cardigans with zippers, Velcro-strap shoes.

o o o

Dressing: Wears the Same Clothes Over and Over

My father had always been a careful dresser. After he retired from his life of white shirts and ties, he wore a full rainbow of golf shirts and owned more cardigans than Mister Rogers. But if you'd met him late in his dementia, you'd invariably see him in a stained plaid shirt and baggy, wrinkled gray trousers—day after day after day.

"The worst part was trying to wash them," recalls my sister-in-law. "He wouldn't put them in the hamper. He hung them up and put them on again in the morning before I could sneak in and get them away." —P.S.S.

WHY it happens:

Impaired short-term memory causes someone with dementia to forget the clothes are dirty as soon as they undress. Impaired judgment means that the usual clues (stained, wrinkled, smelly) don't add up to the usual response (put them in the hamper to be washed).

Donning the same handy clothes the next day is easier than having to choose among many clothes in drawers or the closet. Making choices can be cognitively overwhelming. Familiarity, in contrast, is comforting.

TRY this:

- **Steer clear of logic, such as pointing out, "Honestly, Dad! You wore the same outfit yesterday!"** Not only is it hard for someone with dementia to follow logic but you risk putting him on the defensive and setting up a no-win argument.

- **When the person with dementia is sound asleep, go in his room to remove the dirty clothes**. Lay out something similar in the same spot. As long as replacement clothes are handy in the morning, he's apt to forget about the dirty favorite. If he should notice, make a big fuss over a white lie: "Oh Dad! I'm so sorry! I spilled juice on your favorite shirt yesterday and nearly ruined it! I've sent it to the cleaners, but meanwhile I found this one. Oh, I hope you can forgive me!"

- **Pare down the closet, so there are far fewer options**. Having just a few shirts, for example, can make choosing clean clothes easier. Bonus: If you make sure everything coordinates, there will be no more clashing outfits. Choose solids in a favorite color over patterns, which can be distracting and irritating to someone with dementia.

- **Buy identical multiple versions of favorites**, so one set can be washed while the other is worn. Bonus: Only one type of sock, for example, means no more mismatches or lost mates.

- **If the person sleeps in the same clothes, your only chance may be to take them away for washing when he or she bathes**. Bring clean clothes into the bathroom to put on afterward. You may have to settle for a change of clothes only every few days if daily bathing isn't in the cards.

To help you cope:

- **Make sure the real problem is dirt and odor, not your own irritation by the repetition of the outfit**. A few generations ago, nobody changed clothes every day.

o o o

Dental-Care Trouble

One day Vicki was startled to see her husband, Charles, brushing his teeth with the wrong end of the toothbrush. "What are you doing?" she asked.

"What does it look like?!"

"You're holding the brush upside down!" she told him.

Charles stared at the brush for a second. "I knew that!" he said, putting it down quickly. After that incident, Vicki began to notice that the toothbrush went unused for days.

WHY it happens:

Oral-care problems are common in people with dementia. This is such a central part of private self-care that caregivers sometimes forget about it. We just expect that it's being taken care of, until bad breath, tooth pain, or other problems crop up. Certain medications can cause dry mouth, which interferes with the fit of dentures.

Some people simply forget to brush (or take care of dentures). Others begin having trouble with the steps involved. They may fail to recognize the toothbrush or how to use it, or put shaving cream on the brush instead of toothpaste. Some people swallow mouthwash instead of swishing and spitting.

Getting the person to the dentist for care can be another challenge. Some people grow resistant to doctors, especially a specialist seen only once or twice a year. They may have trouble understanding what's being done to them or why it's important.

TRY this:

- **Brush together**. Sometimes copying a basic task is the easiest way to get it done (and you don't have to make a big deal about reminding). Obviously, this is easier for couples than, say, a parent and child.

- **Set the brush, already loaded with toothpaste, on the sink**. The visual prompt may lead to the task getting done.

- **Break verbal prompts into small steps**: "Pick up the brush. Put it in your mouth. Now brush it against the top teeth," and so on.

- **Although brushing teeth after meals is ideal, this can be taxing even for healthy people**. You might have better luck doing so in the mornings or whenever the person in a good mood. Waiting until evening, when he's tired, can make things harder.

- **For those having trouble identifying personal-care items, consider removing things that might be swallowed or misused**. Mouthwash is a common example.

- **The right tools can help**: Choose a soft brush. A thick handle is easier for many people to hold. Look for brushes designed for children that lack the cartoon characters or other juvenile elements. Some people prefer an electric toothbrush.

- **To brush someone's teeth, seat them in a chair, with head tilted back, and stand behind**. It's okay to use a dry toothbrush and a just a small dot of toothpaste. Offer liquid to rinse after. (It's okay if it's swallowed, if you haven't used much paste.) Or skip toothpaste altogether if it's a problem. Dentists recommend flossing the teeth of people with dementia, but for most people, this rightly falls in the category of way-more-hassle-than-it's-worth.

- **Consult a dentist if you think mouth pain is interfering with oral care**. Before dental exams, make sure the dentist and hygienist are aware of the dementia before they treat your loved one. Bring a list of all medications taken. For troublesome cases, you might want to consider a dentist who specializes in dementia patients; it's a small but growing specialty. (To find one, search on "Alzheimer's" and "dentist" and your zip code or town.) Note that over time, some people lose the ability to tolerate their dentures.

o o o

Grooming Trouble (Hairstyling, Make-Up, and Shaving)

Frank was never one to pay attention to his wife's make-up. All he knew is that Jackie always looked nice. She was a woman who liked to "pretty-up" for him, as he called it. True, her lipstick started to miss her lips a little bit, but he let it go. It made her happy to paint her face.

It rankled when his daughter pulled him aside to say, "Dad! Mom's starting to look like a clown! You can't let her go out like that!"

WHY it happens:

Personal grooming becomes a challenge for many reasons. A person may:

- Skip one or more grooming tasks out of forgetfulness

- Become unable to manage the complicated steps involved

- No longer identify the tools involved (comb, razor, lipstick) and how they're used

Minor grooming mistakes—where someone just looks "off"—are a common early sign of cognitive problems. When awareness is still good in the disease's early stage, the person may realize something's not right or be dissatisfied when grooming no longer comes out the way she'd like. She may redouble her efforts (sometimes making things worse) or begin to avoid them entirely.

TRY this:

Makeup:

- **Avoid embarrassing your loved one with outright criticism**. Aim to correct only in the mildest, most respectful terms, the way you might discreetly point out that someone has spinach in her teeth, for example.

- **Make it easier**. Consider shopping together for (or presenting as a gift or a replacement) lighter shades that are more forgiving of errors in application. Or pitch their other virtues, like a new sheer gloss "that will make your lips feel soft."

- **Casually offer help**: "Here, maybe I can try that?" Or, "Want another pair of hands?"

- **Use process of elimination**. If certain kinds of makeup are really becoming a problem, you might "lose" them and see if they're missed.

Hair:

- **Acknowledge efforts**: "Your hair looks so nice today." Pat a stray piece into place while you say it, if needed.

- **Let the stylist or barber know the person has dementia when you book an appointment**. Ask them to allow for extra time if you think it's needed. Even better, ask a salon if they know any stylists who make house calls— a huge hassle-saver.

- **Go short**. Shorter cuts mean there's less to mess.

- **Move away from an elaborate hairstyle**. Many older women are used to a dye and a permanent wave, which is hard to maintain. As time goes on, it will also be harder to make regular appointments. Discreetly ask the stylist to "accidentally" cut hair extra-short, so you can go longer between trimmings. Exception: A woman who has a long tradition of a weekly salon visit may get pleasure in continuing this social activity. But don't keep it up for her out of loyalty once she no longer seems interested.

- **Ask the stylist to shampoo hair first**. A professional cleaning and conditioning will feel good and be one less time you need to do it.

- **Skip hair products (spray, gel, pomade, dye)**. Simplify. If you stop providing them—"Gee, Mom, you're out"—eventually she'll forget them.

Shaving

- **Set the stage**. Prep the razor and lotion and give simple prompts at each step.

- **Try an electric razor**. It's less likely to nick. Some caregivers report fewer nicks (and fewer steps) with manual razors that have soap built into the cartridge.

Tip: **"My husband usually misses the whiskers on his neck. I make a joke and say, 'Oh, thanks, I see you left a little for me to do for you.'" —A.H.**

- Encourage a man with dementia to quit shaving and grow a beard. Compliment the rugged good look.

To help you cope:

- **Know that grooming deficits can be hard on caregivers because they're a visual reminder that all's not really well.** Even when we tell ourselves that appearances shouldn't matter in the big scheme of things, it can tug at the heart a little.

Tip: **"It sounds corny, but a smile on Momma's face makes her look pretty to me, so that cancels out the goofy hair and the drawn-on crooked eyebrows. Now that's what I aim for, to get her to smile." —C.D.**

o o o

EATING CHALLENGES

Doesn't Eat, Won't Eat

Every afternoon, Gloria dropped off a hot meal for her father, who lived five minutes away. She also made sure his cupboards were stocked with cereal, fresh milk, and sandwich fixings for other meals. He'd never been much of a cook, and since her mother died, she wanted to be sure he ate well.

Lately she'd found the portions untouched. "Pops! Didn't you like the supper?" she'd ask, noticing lots of leftovers from the portions she'd bring him.

The time he ignored the lasagna was the last straw. "Your favorite! Aren't you feeling well?" That's when she began to look more closely into the refrigerator and cupboards. More often than not, she found the milk spoiled, the sandwich meat unopened. He ate heartily at her house but not in his own.

WHY it happens:

Not eating is a common problem that can have many different causes, from situational ones that are easily fixed to some you can't. These include:

- *Cognitive challenges.* Someone who lives alone may find it too difficult to prepare food or even to deal with the sequence of steps involved with realizing it's time for a meal and heating up food that's been prepared in advance—even though he's hungry.

- *Sensory changes.* People with Alzheimer's often have an impaired sense of smell. Aging generally can alter the senses of smell and taste, affecting appetite.

- *Difficulty manipulating utensils.* Holding spoons and forks, filling them with food, and guiding them into the mouth becomes too hard.

- *Not recognizing hunger.* People with dementia can lose touch with bodily functions and what they mean.

- *Inactivity.* People who don't move around much eat less.

- *A physical problem.* Don't overlook causes unrelated to dementia, including a sore mouth, an upset stomach or other illness, a reaction to a new medication, or a problem with the fit of dentures, for example.

- End-stage disease. At the end of life, the body's systems start to shut down and loss of appetite is a natural part of this process. Those with Alzheimer's often have great difficulty swallowing at this point, as well.

TRY this:

- **Use clues about the situation to help pinpoint a cause**. Is the person with dementia losing weight? Is this a sudden change? Are there other signs of illness? Does it happen occasionally (finicky at certain meals) or at most meals? Your exact approach will depend on the likely cause or causes.

- **If you're at all concerned about weight loss or other physical factors affecting eating,** check in with a doctor. Many medications can interfere with appetite.

- **Reassess how the person is getting food**. Is someone available to prepare and serve every meal, or has he been doing some of this on his own? Is he's preparing meals on his own, is he struggling with this responsibility? It's possible more help is now needed. Look into Meals on Wheels or other local agencies that can deliver a daily hot meal.

- **Tilt toward high-caloric, nutrition-dense foods with a birdlike eater**. Good choices include dishes made with cheese, butter, nut butter, eggs, whole milk, crème fraiche, sour cream, and cream. Casseroles (especially made with recipes from older cookbooks) are often heavy on these ingredients. Shakes and smoothies made with fruit and whole milk Greek yogurt, whole milk ice cream, or whole milk are also good.

- **Try strongly flavored foods**. Because taste buds dull for many people as they age, using more herbs, onion, garlic, or other seasonings may make food more appealing.

- **Ask the doctor if the situation makes sense for nutrition drinks that add calories, such as Ensure or Boost**. They're not intended for use as meal replacements, but as supplements between meals. If you use them, be sure to include mention of them when doctors ask which medications and supplements the person is taking.

- **Offer snacks throughout the day**, such as high-calorie energy bars, oatmeal cookies, yogurt. Some people who tend to avoid big meals will willingly take a few bites if offered.

- **Be aware that trouble managing a fork, knife, and spoon can be embarrassing to the point of limiting intake**. Different kinds of foods or utensils can sidestep this issue. See also in this chapter: "Messy Eating."

- **Never force-feed**. No matter how good your intentions, it can be traumatic and is often counterproductive.

- **Consider periodically weighing the person if you're alarmed about weight loss**. Losing a lot of weight in a short time is a key thing doctors look for when deciding if someone is a candidate for hospice. If you can show this change, it might be easier to get the person enrolled.

What About Feeding Tubes?

Don't assume that tube feeding (supplying liquid nutrition through a tube inserted into the throat or abdomen) is the most humane option when someone with dementia shows little interest in eating. There's been a strong movement away from this method of treating people with advanced Alzheimer's because it often does more harm than good. Caregivers tend to have high expectations for this treatment, according to an *Archives of Internal Medicine* study. But this study and others have found those hopes are rarely met.

Research shows that for those with advanced dementia, tube feeding doesn't increase weight, improve nutrition, improve strength, or help prevent aspiration pneumonia. Surprisingly, it doesn't even extend life. Feeding tubes tend to cause diarrhea and discomfort and increase the risk of infection and pressure sores, while distancing the person from human touch. Unable to understand what the tube is for (or forgetting), some people with Alzheimer's try to pull it out. The next step in some medical care is to tie the hands down or give sedatives.

The Alzheimer's Association's official position: "It is ethically permissible to withhold nutrition and hydration artificially administered by vein or gastric tube when the person with Alzheimer's disease or dementia is in the end stages of the disease and is no longer able to receive food or water by mouth."

Consult with medical staff and hospice professionals if you face this very difficult juncture. Know that it tends to be much harder to get a feeding tube removed than to have it placed, due to organizational policies, especially in the absence of an advance directive about life support. They're designed for short-term use for someone who's recovering from a stroke or surgery and is expected to improve.

The more compassionate alternative when someone can't eat: hand feeding ice chips and any food that will be taken (called assisted oral feeding). Don't fear that your loved one is "starving to death" as this is not what's happening in this situation. The body is already shutting down by natural process. Without food or water, the body releases endorphins, a substance that blunts pain. (See Chapter 5: "End-of-Life Care.")

o o o

Forgets Having Eaten, Wants More

One hot summer day, I cubed a big bowl of watermelon for my dad. "Thank you!" he said, digging in as he watched his baseball game.

I returned to the kitchen to finish the dishes and cut up some more fruit for myself.

"For me?" Dad said, pleased, as I entered the family room.

I was confused but handed him the bowl, figuring he was still hungry. My mother shouted from across the room in exasperation. "You just ate some!" To me, she said, "He does this all the time, lately!"

Dad didn't seem to recognize that the empty bowl beside him had been his. Whether you walked in with a bowl of watermelon, ice cream, nuts, popcorn—and whether or not he'd just polished off his own bowl—when Dad saw food while he was watching sports, that was action he wanted a piece of. —P.S.S.

WHY it happens:

An eroding short-term memory makes it hard for someone with dementia to remember what just happened. Add to this an inability to read the body's signals, such as hunger or satiety. When my dad sat down to watch a ballgame, this was the trigger for him to want to eat. Boredom can add to a desire to find pleasure in food.

Someone who says, "I'm hungry" may also be expressing (without fully realizing it) a hunger of a different sort—for attention, for affection, for something to do.

TRY this:

- **Sidestep arguments or logic**. ("But you just ate!") Someone with Alzheimer's at this stage can't follow a rational argument.

- **Within reason, go ahead and offer the requested food if it's reasonably harmless**. Tread more carefully with empty calories that can cause mood to crash or spoil the person's appetite for meals, if that's an issue.

- **Offer a hug and a distracting conversation**: "Oh, we're all out of that. But let's plan the perfect dinner, and I'll shop later."

- **Try breaking up the meal**. Serve half now, half later. Or serve eggs and toast at breakfast, followed by fruit and yogurt for successive snacks.

- **Offer a snack "to tide you over until it's ready."** Something light might avoid an argument and make someone forget about wanting another full meal.

- **Maybe just don't sit there after dinner**. Try to engage an ever-hungry person in a busy post-meal activity to distract him, like a walk or something involving the hands.

o o o

Gets Distracted During Meals

Elena usually comes to the table in a docile, agreeable way. But getting her to eat the meal can be vexing to her daughter, Maria. Elena goes through the right motions at the start. She puts her napkin in her lap, says a blessing, picks up her fork, and says, every time, "Why this looks delicious, dear."

But somewhere after the first forkful, Elena seems to forget why she's there. Her bites seem to slow down, and her attention wanders. As Maria's family talks about the day and gobbles down the meal, Elena often simply shuts down.

"Mama, eat!" Maria says every few minutes. Elena smiles, takes a bite...and then stops again.

WHY it happens:

A frustratingly slow, indifferent eater isn't purposely annoying you. She can't help it. Think about the sheer number of steps involved with eating: recognizing hunger, connecting it to the food before you, choosing to pick up a fork and fill it with one of the choices on your plate, and then bringing the forkful to your mouth to chew and swallow. At every step, competing interests, such as conversation, background noise, the various bowls or flowers on the table, can distract and slow the process.

Some people enter a stage of playing with their food. They simply forget what the food is or what should be done with it.

TRY this:

- **Help direct focus to the plate**. Remove clutter from the table: papers, books, knick-knacks, centerpiece, napkin holders, salt and pepper shakers.

- **Turn off the TV and talk radio**. Soft music may help set a positive mood or be too distracting; experiment.

- **Highlight the plate and cup by placing them on a contrasting placement**. Use a white plate on a blue mat, say. A study in *Clinical Nutrition* found that people with Alzheimer's eat more when using high-contrast tableware.

- **Avoid patterned dishes and table coverings**. Solids are best because patterns can disorient or distract. Solid cups are less distracting than glass ones, through which liquid and distortion can be seen.

- **Use fewer utensils**. If only a fork is needed, don't set out knives and spoons. One utensil for the whole meal is fine. A spork (combination spoon and fork) works double-duty and is often easier for someone with trembly hands to manage. Metal is safer than plastic, which can be accidentally bitten off and swallowed.

- **Put one or two foods on the plate at a time**, in small, manageable servings. You can always add more after it's eaten. A plateful of different choices may overwhelm.

- **Make sure foods aren't too hot**. The diner may lose interest while waiting for something to cool.

- **Offer calm, casual prompts through the meal**. This is especially useful with someone who stops eating or plays with food (usually in later stages of the disease). "Pick up your fork...scoop the beans...take a bite...now swallow...isn't it good?" Better to encourage self-feeding than to do it for someone, if they're physically capable of the mechanics.

- **Use positive reinforcement before and during the meal so good feelings are linked to the sight of the table**. Talk about the delicious meal you're about to have, how good it smells. End on a positive note with a favorite dessert, even something as simple as a few cookies.

- **Avoid rushing the person**. The whole table doesn't have to eat courses in unison. Put all the food out at once. If kids eat fast and finish early, excuse them rather than having them fidget and add tension.

To help you cope:

- **Separate food from love in your mind**. That's difficult for most of us, having been raised from childhood to find pleasure or reward in a cookie or to bask in pride when guests praise our dishes. Your loved one may still enjoy food, and yours in particular, but the disease can make it impossible to express this through words or deeds.

o o o

Messy Eating

I winced as Dad bit into the hot dog. Sure enough, big droplets of ketchup and mustard landed on his clean chinos. His napkin had already fluttered from his lap. Crumbs from the bun floated down next, landing in the sticky liquids. As usual, he seemed not to notice.

Half of every handful of potato chips made it into his mouth. The rest smashed against his cheek and crumbled to his lap. Too late, I replaced the napkin. I dabbed a ketchup blot from his lips. When he lifted a can of soda, I knew before it happened that at least some of the cola would dribble across his shirt.

Overall, the picnic was a success. Dad ate a full meal, and he enjoyed listening to the live band and watching the grandchildren race around. But my sister's kindergartener went home cleaner than Grandpa did. —P.S.S.

WHY it happens:

Cognitive and physical changes combine to make it difficult to eat neatly. Some people lose some fine-motor control (over hands, utensils) and hand-eye coordination, either due to the dementia or another condition. At the same time, they tend to become less attentive to what they're doing or where the stray food bits are going. They may be oblivious about mess, both during the meal and after.

TRY this:

- **Lower your expectations and look the other way as much as you can**. Spills can be mopped. Clothes can be washed.

- **Make sure the fit between chair and table is snug**. Some chairs have heavy arms that don't fit under the table, so food must travel a little farther to get to the mouth. Swap in a chair that fits.

- **Unobtrusively place a napkin in your loved one's lap before serving food if he no longer does this himself**. It might not stay there, but it's a start. Cloth napkins mean more laundry but tend to stay in place better than paper.

- **Cut up foods before serving them in manageable, bite-sized pieces**. It can feel infantilizing to have the food on your plate cut for you, so either cut all the food before placing it in the serving dish or plate the food before you bring it to the table.

- **To ease cleanup, try a vinyl tablecloth**. They're more easily wiped clean. Or use paper placemats that can be thrown away.

- **Serve fewer messy foods**. The most problematic have sauces and condiments (mustard, ketchup, mayo). Pre-season food before bringing it to the table.

- **Switch to a "spork"—a combination spoon and fork—if manipulating utensils is difficult**. They're sold in camping stores or online. Spoons are generally easier than forks, and anything with a thick handle is easier to grip.

- **Try serving food in a bowl instead of a plate**. Bowls better contain mess. Look for shallow, rimmed pasta dishes, which seem plate-like.

- **Serve finger foods**. No-utensils-necessary examples: fried chicken or fish, chicken strips, shrimp, pizza cut into bite-sized squares, fish sticks, bacon, and unadorned vegetables such as green beans, corn on the cob, diced squash, sweet potato fries, or roasted cubes of potato. Cook eggs omelet-style firm and cut them into strips or squares that can be picked up. Try foods in "edible wrappers" including finger sandwiches, spring rolls, pita pockets, won tons, dumplings, pierogi, tacos, fajitas, and the like.

- **At first, offer the finger-food and bite-sized meals to everyone at the table**. The messy eater won't feel singled out. Later, he or she may not notice.

- **Serve soup in a mug**. That way it can be sipped, rather than using a bowl and spoon. Let it cool a bit first.

- **Try a lidded cup with a spout for liquids**. They're sold in hospital-supply stores. If you use a regular cup, pour it only about one third full.

- **Use the most solid dishes you have**. Think heavy ironstone rather than fine china or thin melamine. Dishes with heft will be less likely to slip around.

- **Choose heavy plastic cups over glass ones if grip is a problem**. Solid colors are better than transparent glass, which can be disorienting to look through, adding to spills.

- **Use bigger-sized napkins**. Someone in the later stages might consent to wearing a smock apron during meals.

- **Keep the tone pleasant**. If you need to point out a mistake (mustard smeared on the cheek, for example), do so in a casual way: "Oh that mustard got on you, too. Here, let me get it."

Tip: **"I bought a food grinder to turn meals into finger-friendly options, like meatballs or meat and vegetables I'd put in puff pastry." —A.A.**

o o o

Won't Drink Enough Liquids

Emma broke her wrist in a nighttime fall while still in her early 60s. Ever since, she'd been careful not to drink much in the evenings, so she wouldn't have to get up to go to the bathroom. As she got older and her bladder weakened, she'd begun avoiding liquids in the afternoons, too.

As her dementia progressed, Emma forgot many things. But the habit of not drinking liquids seemed to intensify. She refused anything to drink at any time of day. Her exasperated sister, Mary, was able to get her to take just a few sips with her pills but little more.

WHY it happens:

People with dementia may not get enough liquids for a variety of reasons:

- Often they lose the ability to "read" the sensation of thirst. Also adults tend to feel less thirst generally as they age.

- They may be thirsty but not express it.

- They may simply forget to take sips along with meals or snacks during the day.

- They may avoid drinking, as Emma does, because they want to avoid the effects of liquids—having to get up to use the bathroom or difficulty in undressing and getting there in time. Some people want to avoid using the bathroom in public and will avoid drinking if they have to go to a doctor appointment or somewhere else.

The key risk to not drinking enough liquids is dehydration. It's a real risk among older adults with dementia, especially when the weather is warm or when taking medications that are dehydrating. A good idea: Ask the doctor whether dehydration is a side effect of any meds on the list of the person in your care, so you can know whether this is an issue to look out for.

TRY this:

- **Offer liquids throughout the day**. Don't wait for the person with dementia to ask for a drink. Aim for 6-8 total cups of fluid a day.

- **Don't just hand over a glass**. Stand by and make sure the drink is actually sipped.

- **Issue mild prompts during the meal**: "Have a sip of water, Sis. Try the iced tea."

- **Vary the types of beverages offered**: water, iced tea, juice, milk, hot chocolate, cider. Even coffee and soda are okay in moderation (about a cup a day) if they're preferred. The latest thinking is that a cup or two a day doesn't pose a diuretic effect that would lead to dehydration. For someone not consuming enough liquids, liquids in any form are probably beneficial.

- **Do, however, curb caffeinated beverages if fear of getting to the bathroom on time is an issue**. Caffeinated drinks can cause frequent urination. Also avoid them if sleep is already a problem.

- **Leave water bottles around the house where the person likes to sit**. Many older adults aren't in the habit of drinking this way, though, so if it doesn't work, don't press the point.

- **Serve liquidy foods to make up some of the total**. Fruit contains a lot of water, especially watermelon, cantaloupe, honeydew, grapes, and citrus. Soup or broth is another option.

- **For a liquid refusenik, invoke the doctor**: "He wants you to drink this." Or, "She says this much is okay."

- **For someone worried about getting to the bathroom on time, don't wait for him or her to need to go**. Make the suggestion 20 to 30 minutes after drinking something. It's a relief to everyone when clothes are easy-on, easy-off, such as pants with elastic waistbands and no belt.

- **Learn the symptoms of dehydration**: increased confusion or lethargy, complaints of headache or dizziness, dry skin or mouth, unusually yellowish or dark urine, skin that feels warm to the touch. Call the doctor, who may recommend a rehydration solution (such as Pedialyte). If you can't rehydrate the person by getting her to take liquids and you don't see a change in symptoms, she may need IV (intravenous) hydration.

Diarrhea and vomiting increase the risk of dehydration, so monitor closely, and notify the doctor if you suspect dehydration.

o o o

HEALTH CHALLENGES

Confusion That Worsens Suddenly (Delirium)

Maria had to be hospitalized overnight when she'd begun to complain about chest pain, and family members were concerned an old heart valve replacement was no longer working well. Her daughter Aurelia stayed with her, catnapping on an easy chair next to the bed. A little after midnight, Maria awakened, asking where her husband, Luis, was. Luis had died almost eight years earlier. At first Aurelia wasn't too concerned. Her mom sometimes forgot he'd died, and often mixed up lots of other dates and facts as her Alzheimer's had worsened.

But then Maria began to babble in Spanish. Though fluent, Aurelia could nevertheless make out only bits and pieces because her mother was talking so fast and yet in fragments. Maria seemed to be talking about flying over fields of corn looking for Luis. She heard her comment how pretty the sunshine was, how much she enjoyed flying, and how they had to get home before her father caught them.

"Then she started to grow more agitated, clutching at the bed sheets and calling everybody's name: Luis! Papa! Aurelia! All of us mixed together. It almost sounded like a dream, but she was wide awake," Aurelia says. "And she would not respond to me or focus on me.

"It was very scary and went on for some time."

Aurelia was sure that just being in the hospital had caused her mom's Alzheimer's to worsen. Then she found out that her mother had developed a urinary tract infection, quite separate from the heart issue. After a week on antibiotics, Maria seemed to return to the way she was before the hospitalization.

WHY it happens:

Delirium—a reversible state of acute mental confusion—is usually caused by a stress that affects the whole body. The stress could be any number of things:

- a known or new infection (like pneumonia, UTI, or a skin infection)

- low oxygen level (brought on by heart attack or a lung exacerbation from COPD)

- a medication reaction

- sleep deprivation

- pain

- dehydration

- acute emotional stress, including depression or a psychiatric condition

Hospitalization itself is a huge risk factor for delirium. One 2013 study found that more than half of all people with dementia who are hospitalized will experience delirium. The risk is also higher when someone in the hospital is dehydrated, an alcoholic, or undergoing anesthesia.

Delirium isn't a disease; it's a syndrome of changes caused by an underlying problem. As brain function is scrambled due to the delirium, it causes behaviors that are sometimes your only clue to a life-threatening illness. That's why it's important for a family caregiver to be able to recognize it. Doctors and nurses often miss it because they don't know your loved one as well as you do—and tend to attribute what they're seeing to the fact that the person has dementia.

The signs of delirium vary from person to person. There's no single way someone acts delirious. So trust your intuition. When a caregiver senses something's "off" about a family member's behavior or functioning, there's often a very real reason for it.

Here are the most common signs of delirium in someone with dementia:

- *A sudden turn for the worse in the usual state of mental impairment.* The change usually happens over a period of hours but sometimes comes on more gradually (over days). Look for a change in what's normal for that person (whatever his or her current, demented "normal" is).

- *Fluctuating confusion.* A tricky aspect of delirium is that the mental changes in awareness and orientation come and go. The person may alternate between seeming fine at moments and seeming much more confused than usual at other times. The person probably already has good days and bad days, or good and bad times of day. So how can you identify changes associated with delirium? The problem is similar to that of parents trying to assess whether a child is truly sick versus just having a fussy day. Look for deviations from usual behavior or patterns in a typical day. Many people with dementia ordinarily have better mornings than late afternoons, for example. In that case, extra confusion that appears in the morning might be a red flag.

- *Difficulty paying attention.* The person has trouble focusing (on conversation, on anything).

- *Agitation, being more revved up than usual.* This can range from a surge in nervous energy to increased combativeness or anger. Someone who's usually mild-mannered may behave aggressively.

- *Acting much quieter or drowsier.* Although "being delirious" tends to call up images of raving madness, in many people delirium manifests as becoming quieter and more spaced out. This is called hypoactive delirium and is just as dangerous.

- *Hallucinations/delusions.* The person doesn't act like his or her usual self. He or she may see or hear things that aren't real, make false accusations, or otherwise not be grounded in reality. In someone with dementia who already has been having hallucinations or delusions, they may be more frequent or troubling.

Once you notice the first possible signs of delirium, pay even closer attention to other possible changes over the next hours and days. And be prepared to act quickly if you do see signs.

Why the urgency? For a condition that many laypeople have never even heard of, delirium can be catastrophic to someone with dementia. Some people come out of it with a lower level of cognitive functioning then they had and never recover to their old baseline. Others decline as much as twice as rapidly in the months following a bout of delirium.

TRY this:

After you notice signs of delirium:

- **Start with a medical evaluation, quickly**. If you're at home, call 911 or go to the emergency room if you notice signs of delirium and there's also been a serious fall, a head injury or broken bone, or the person is having trouble staying conscious or breathing. If these crisis signs don't apply, it's still a good idea to get an urgent-care appointment with the person's primary care provider if you can.

- **If you're already in a hospital, alert staff**. Let them know you suspect delirium and why. Fast action matters because, while there's no drug that treats delirium, the treatment is usually a matter of identifying and treating the underlying cause. Once this happens, the delirium usually improves in a matter of hours or days, although in elderly adults it can take weeks or even months to get back to their best mental selves.

- **Don't count on hospital staff to notice delirium**. It can be hard to identify in someone who "normally" has confusion and memory loss. Trust your instincts. You know your loved one's current status better than anyone. Be persistent about pointing out what seems different so it doesn't get written off as "but she has dementia." You'd be surprised how often even doctors and nurses fail to recognize delirium in patients, especially in those who already have Alzheimer's or other forms of dementia.

- **Stay with the person during an evaluation**. You have to be there to express what's typical and answer any questions.

- **Bring all medications to an evaluation**. That includes prescriptions; over-the-counter drugs for pain, colds, and allergies; and nutritional supplements. These are a common cause or contributor to delirium. Don't forget medications that were started and stopped for any reason or that recently ran out or ended.

- **Pay attention to the work-up for delirium**. A good doctor will investigate possible underlying causes by doing a physical exam (looking for fever and other signs of infection, for example, and taking vital signs and possibly ordering blood or urine tests). Pain will also be assessed, such as following a fall or from constipation. People with Alzheimer's often fail to report their pain, so the doctor can't rely on the person's word on this. Finally, the work-up should include a medications review.

To prevent delirium:

- **Think carefully about whether a recommended surgery is absolutely necessary for someone with dementia**. Also avoid elective surgeries or any procedures involving sedation, if you possibly can. The risk of worsening dementia afterward is real and big.

- **If your loved one must ever be hospitalized, arrange for someone to stay with him or her** throughout the stay, 24/7—if you possibly can. Someone with any degree of cognitive impairment is unable to keep track of what doctors say and do, much less speak up for herself about her symptoms and needs. Moreover, a hospital can be a distressing and disorienting place for someone with Alzheimer's. Your steady, familiar presence can go a long way to reducing stress. You'll also be able to identify signs of delirium (as Aurelia noticed with her mother) and can alert hospital staff.

- **If you have the option, look for a hospital with an acute-care-for-elders unit**. These typically minimize sleep disruptions, avoid physical restraints, and take other steps to avoid stressors that can lead to delirium.

- **In the hospital, make sure the person has glasses, hearing aids, dentures, and other assistive devices handy as needed**. They're often taken off for sleep or a procedure, and in the hospital hubbub, not returned—contributing to disorientation. You know what your family member uses; the night nurse doesn't. Provide extra orienting reminders: "You're in the hospital to have your heart checked." Say it over and over. Don't be shy about asking medical staff what can be done to ensure that the person gets enough to drink (to avoid dehydration) and gets enough sleep (especially at night, when checks and medication dispensing can disorient someone with Alzheimer's).

- **Pay attention to hydration**. Even healthy older adults tend to drink less liquid than they should. Older adults with dementia can simply forget and lose the ability to read their body's signals for thirst. This can worsen in hot weather or when someone's feeling under the weather. In the study that showed half of all hospitalized dementia patients experience delirium, one third of these patients were found to be dehydrated on admittance (though that wasn't the reason for the hospitalization).

By some estimates, nearly half of delirium cases in hospitals can be eliminated through steps like these.

o o o

Constipation

Gerald didn't seem like himself. He moaned a lot. But he couldn't exactly say what was wrong. His wife, Gloria, felt his forehead— no fever. She put her hands on his arms and legs, but he didn't seem to have any tender spots. He didn't flinch when she touched his back and knees, places where his arthritis had always been most severe. But he wouldn't stop moaning.

Then he didn't even want to eat. Alarmed, she took him to the doctor.

Gerald's arthritis is severe enough that he starting taking a prescription pain reliever several months ago. It's helped the pain but has had an often-unrecognized side effect. It causes constipation.

WHY it happens:

Constipation is defined as having pain or difficulty emptying the bowels, or straining for several minutes, usually due to hard stool. As a rule of thumb, going three days without a bowel movement (BM) is a flag for constipation. In general, the goal is to have a comfortable BM every one to two days.

Alzheimer's isn't normally a cause (constipation can happen to anyone), but people with Alzheimer's do have a few added strikes against them:

- They tend to lose the ability to read their body's signals. Unable to know when they're hungry or thirsty, they're at higher risk of dehydration, which can cause constipation. They also may not be aware when they need to use the bathroom.

- They have a hard time articulating pain of impacted BMs.

- They often become less active and sit more, raising the risk.

- They may be prescribed anticholinergics (including Benadryl and/or narcotic pain relievers), which raise the risk.

- People with non-Alzheimer's dementias such as Parkinson's or Lewy Body can develop constipation when the nerves of the digestive system are affected.

- The incidence of constipation rises with age.

Untreated, constipation can darken mood and escalate behavior problems. Chronic constipation can also lead to fecal impaction, in which feces stuck in the bowels causes other health problems. People who use laxatives for a long time are at added risk of this.

"Constipation is considered a less-than-glamorous topic by doctors, but proper treatment can make a world of difference to an older patient," says San Francisco geriatrician Leslie Kernisan.

TRY this:

To prevent constipation problems:

- **In general, offer plenty of liquids**. Remember, it doesn't have to be water. Also good: soup, pulpy orange juice, thinned hot cereal (such as diluted Cream of Wheat), frozen fruit bars, lemonade.

- **Serve a diet that includes plant foods and whole-grain fiber**. Realize, though, that certain medications will create a tendency to constipation regardless of a healthy diet.

- **Encourage movement**. Consider this yet another reason for your loved one to walk around and have other physical activity each day.

- **Watch for facial grimaces that come out of the blue**. Listen for grunting or other signs of pain when the person uses the toilet. You might catch on early to a case of constipation, so it can be treated.

- **Don't obsess over BMs**. Not everyone goes every day. But if you're so inclined, to prevent a repeat episode it can help to track toileting habits so you have a sense when it's been awhile and notice other symptoms (such as grimacing or pain).

To treat constipation:

- **Talk to the doctor about the best option to get things moving**. There are many options, and some can be bought at your local drugstore. But they each have their pros and cons. Be sure to mention to the doctor whether you're dealing with acute or chronic constipation. Acute constipation (a specific current episode) requires something to get the person unplugged. Many older adults are chronically a bit constipated and need to figure out what kind of regimen will keep them regular.

- **Ask about the options**. Dr. Kernisan notes that the four main types of laxatives used for constipation are:

1. Osmotic agents (laxatives with non-absorbable sugars) to draw water into the bowel. This makes stool softer. Prune juice is one choice. The over-the-counter drug MiraLax is another. There are also prescription alternatives.

2. Stimulating agents to act directly on the colon stimulate the muscles. The OTC agent senna is one choice, or a suppository may be prescribed.

3. Softening agents to make the stool softer and more slippery. The best known and most prescribed is Colace, but it's not as effective as the other choices.

4. Fiber "bulking agents" to bulk up the stool in order to get the colon working right. The OTC powder Metamucil is a popular example. Fiber has to be taken with a lot of water so it doesn't stop things up. And it can cause gas and bloating, so it's not a good choice for everyone.

Sometimes a combination of these is recommended. Dr. Kernisan also emphasizes that many older adults take some laxative every day and that this shouldn't be cause for concern. It's generally safe, and the benefits greatly outweigh the small theoretical risk, she says.

Be wary of lowering pain medication to avoid or lessen constipation. In general, older adults tend to receive too little pain medication, not too much. It's better for the patient to treat the symptom of constipation rather than try to eliminate it by cutting out the pain drug causing it, she suggests.

o o o

Incontinence and Adult "Diapers" *

My grandmother, then in her early 90s and fairly deep in her dementia, was living with my cousin when she began to have "accidents." Not that she drew any attention to them, at least not with her words. Instead she'd remove the wet underpants and carefully set them out to dry...on the radiator. "You'd walk in the front door and—whew! Instant nursing home smell," my cousin recalls.

Once, when nobody was home, she got a large cooking pot from the kitchen, used it as a makeshift commode, and replaced it on its shelf, without a word. —P.S.S.

* NOTE: It's best to avoid using the word "diapers" because it's demeaning and outdated. I've used it here only because this is how people often search for information about incontinence and personal-care products.

WHY it happens:

Incontinence—loss of bladder or bowel control—can be part of the progression of Alzheimer's as well as a result of other problems the person might be having. Any accidents can be dicey to discuss, given the privacy and embarrassment surrounding the issue. An added challenge is that by the time accidents begin, the person is usually deep into the disease and lacks insight and logic.

Someone with Alzheimer's who starts having accidents might hide them, as in my Gram's case. Or she may react obliviously every time. My dad used to try to outsmart the problem by unzipping right in the hallway, all the better to make it to the commode on time (with mixed results). Those who are delusional might try to blame other people: "He threw water on my bed."

Non-Alzheimer's causes, many of which are treatable, can include:

- Chronic urinary issues due to overactive bladder, prostate issues (men), and/or pelvic muscle relaxation (women)
- Urinary tract infections
- Medication reactions
- Certain food or drink triggers (such as colas and caffeine)

TRY this:

- **Start by recognizing that "job one" isn't to get your loved one into wearing incontinence products**. It's to get a doctor to rule out any possible medical problems, especially if the incontinence is new or getting worse. It's always better to address the situation this way rather than avoid it, hoping it will go away. Many causes for incontinence are treatable. You don't have to make a big deal about it as the purpose of a doctor visit if you're worried the person might be embarrassed. Make an appointment on the pretext of something else—a flu shot, say, or a medication check—and alert the staff in advance.

  A bonus with starting with the doctor is that he or she can "prescribe" incontinence products. When a neutral third party recommends them, you don't have to play the bad guy.

- **Have empathy**—even though dealing with this problem can be really, really annoying, especially when it happens for the second or third time in the middle of the night. Someone with dementia isn't "doing it on purpose" or "doing it to get back at you." Loss of bladder control means just that. He or she can't control it.

- **Realize that early in dementia, you're apt to be as uncomfortable talking about the subject as the person having trouble**. Later, it's common to encounter less resistance, though not always. Being matter of fact and approaching it as a health issue, not a personal problem, works best. Humor can help for some: "Well, you finally have something in common with those famous old TV stars on the commercials!"

- **Keep repeating the doctor's advice to use products**. The person with dementia isn't going to remember and needs to be reminded of new behaviors.

- **Show you're on his or her side**: "I know you hate this, but the doctor thinks we can find out why this is happening." "I know it's annoying for you, but the doctor says if we do x and y...." No one likes wetting herself, but everyone tends to feel relieved about the prospect of taking action.

- **Consider a wardrobe change**. Old outfits outlive their usefulness when the goal is getting to the bathroom quickly. Men might be able to skip wearing a belt, for example, or switch to pants with a large zipper. (Skip button flies or overalls!) Both genders often prefer pull-down sweatpants or elastic-waist pants. Women with incontinence do better without stockings.

- **Make the bathroom easy to use**. Among the improvements caregivers report success with: a taller-than-normal commode (easier to sit down on); grab bars near the toilet; a toilet seat in a contrasting color to the commode (a dark seat in a white bathroom to aid depth-perception).

- **Consider a bedside commode**. Trips to the bathroom in the dark and night can be slower than usual. Relocate the wastebasket so it's not mistaken for a commode.

- **Look for cues the person needs to go**. These might be obvious (pulling at pants, wiggling) or more subtle (a certain facial expression or increasing agitation, for example).

- **Listen for special language that refers to the need to use the toilet or to having had an accident**. It's typical to refer to rain or showers, for example.

- **Keep a toileting schedule for a while to track bathroom use and accidents**. You'll probably be able to find a pattern and can lead her to the bathroom in advance.

- **Offer verbal reminders**. Because you can't rely on her body to signal when she needs to use the bathroom, it helps for you to say so: "It's a long drive. Let's go to the bathroom before we go."

- **Let go of your own preconceptions about incontinence products**. The range of options has evolved a lot, and many products resemble underwear. You might be surprised how readily someone takes to them once the fear of accidents is over.

- **If your loved one is resistant to using them, emphasize the advantages**: We'll be able to stay out longer, you can go to your program without embarrassment, you'll feel more comfortable, the modern kind are so good nobody can even tell what they are. Point out how common they are. ("Why do you think they make so many of them?")

- **Watch your language**. Instead of saying *diapers*, use words like *briefs, panties, special pants, protective underwear*, or just *new underpants*.

- **Switch out the old underwear cold turkey, rather than making their use optional**. Someone with dementia might have an easier time getting used to a change when there's no visual reminder of old underwear.

- **Don't stop at undergarments**. Ask the doctor about which lotions, cleansers, and skin barriers would be best to protect an incontinent person's skin. People with bowel and bladder accidents are at a higher risk of bedsores, infections, and other skin problems.

- **Invest in waterproof sheets, bedcovers, and chair pads, too**. Though not inexpensive, they can save you a lot of grief.

- **Be aware that someone with moderate dementia may not be able to identify when an incontinence garment is wet or full**. You may need to double check, or encourage changing on a regular schedule, so the person doesn't keep the same one on all day as if it were actual underwear.

Tip: **"If I say Mom's briefs are 'wet' she gets mad and says 'no they're not.' If I say they look 'heavy,' she'll change right away." —E.L.**

To help you cope:

- **Avoid comparing your situation to others**. You have to do what's best for you on this one. For some caregivers, persistent incontinence ultimately becomes a "deal breaker" that necessitates a move out of a private home. Others find that the problem is manageable and don't mind so much. How you experience it can depend on many factors, including the severity of the problem, whether you're encountering both bowel and bladder incontinence, what kind of help is available, the person's mobility, and your relative sizes (since help with toileting is a physical task).

o o o

Sleeps Too Little, Disturbed Sleep

"Oh no, not again." Rick looked at the clock: 3:15. It was the third time his mother-in-law had been up that night, rapping on their bedroom door. He rolled over and wrapped the pillow over his head.

Carol sighed, too. She couldn't go back to sleep, though. She knew her mother, Betty, would keep on knocking. An hour ago, she'd awakened their teenage son—and he usually slept through anything!

Sometimes Betty simply woke up and rummaged around in her room. If she left the room to use the bathroom, however, all bets were off. She'd travel from the bathroom to the kitchen, see nobody there, and proceed to wander through the house looking for them, until she came to Rick and Carol's locked bedroom door. And the knocking would begin.

At first, when this pattern started, Carol thought her mother needed help in the bathroom. Then she tried soothing her back to sleep with some warm milk and a gentle back rub. Some nights, this did the trick. Other nights, Carol would finally turn on the TV and let her mom fall asleep in front of it, which worked for a few precious hours at a stretch.

WHY it happens:

The effects of Alzheimer's on sleep (and vice versa) aren't fully understood. Because sleep's control centers lie deep within the brain, the changes that occur there due to disease can in turn disrupt the natural rhythms that govern sleep. One common pattern: oversleeping by day, or feeling drowsy during the day, and then feeling more wakeful at night. Alzheimer's medications can disrupt sleep in some people.

What's all too well understood, however, is that disrupted sleep is one of the biggest problems many caregivers face. A live-in loved one's sleep trouble becomes your sleep trouble, too.

Without enough sleep, someone with dementia becomes more irritable, confused, and prone to difficult behaviors. There's an association between lack of sleep and agitated behaviors. Caregivers who function on too-little sleep, in turn, can also experience fuzzy thinking, fatigue, mood changes, weight gain, and more. There's growing evidence that lack of sleep is linked to chronic diseases such as high blood pressure, diabetes, heart disease, and depression—even the development of Alzheimer's itself. So it's a serious matter.

On top of the brain changes of dementia, it's possible that insomnia and restless sleeping are being caused by a factor other than Alzheimer's. These causes might include:

- *Sleep apnea.* This often undiagnosed condition causes a person to stop breathing momentarily. It's very common in people who are overweight, and high-risk groups also include smokers and anyone over 65. Red flags: loud snoring or gasping during sleep.

- *An overactive bladder,* causing night waking or incontinence.

- *Restless legs syndrome.* One in 10 American adults has this tingling sensation that creates a strong urge to keep moving your legs, and the incidence increases with age.

- *Depression.* Sleep disruptions are a major sign of depression, which itself occurs more often in people who have dementia.

- *Medication reactions.* Beta blockers, for example, can cause insomnia, and diuretics can wake you up to relieve your bladder.

- *Pain,* whether from a known or unknown condition.

- *Age.* Adults of all ages need about the same amount of sleep (7 to 8 hours). But sleep cycles change so that an older adult spends more time in light sleep, compared to deep sleep.

These common sleep problems are health threats for anyone. (You may experience some of them yourself.) When you also have dementia, however, it's harder to follow treatments or to self-calm and get back to sleep. For example, someone with dementia is not a prime candidate for a CPAP machine, the breathing-aid device that's the main treatment for sleep apnea. The ensuing agitation and disruption then becomes an issue for the whole household.

Part of the reason the problem is so tough is that a combination of causes (brain changes, other physical causes, depression, medications, age) can all be in play at once.

TRY this:

- **Start with trying to alter behavior or the environment**. Both over-the-counter and prescription sleep medications have many side effects that can backfire, ranging from raising the risk of dangerous falls to increased mortality, so they're considered a last resort. What's more, studies show less effectiveness for the usual sleep aids, such as Ambien, for people with Alzheimer's. Some caregivers report success with the hormone melatonin, but clinical trials have shown no effect, perhaps because people with Alzheimer's have fewer melatonin receptors, according to a Johns Hopkins report.

- **Stick to a predictable daily routine**, in which the day begins and ends at about the same times. Daytime naps should also come at the same time and be about the same length each day.

Review the daily routine:

- **Does it include exposure to sunlight in the morning?** Bright light, soon after waking, can help reset the body's inner clock and encourage sleep later.

- **Is there time to get outside and get some exercise—** even just walking around the house and yard? If you're already taking one walk a day, try taking two.

- **Are naps getting overlong?** Hours of napping midday will interfere with evening sleep.

- **Are meals at about the same time each day?** They're key to a consistent routine.

- **Is the evening wind-down calming?** Dim the lighting when the sun goes down and keep activities after dinner on the quiet side (no loud TV).

- **Do you use the same sleep cues each night when it's time to turn in?** Follow the same series of soothing events nightly. For example, you might shut all the shades, serve a small mug of warm cocoa, assist with brushing teeth and washing up, and play soft classical music in the bedroom.

More things to try:

- **In addition to getting bright morning light, keep the living area bright during the day**. Open curtains, turn on lights on gloomy days, and get outside or encourage sitting near a window. Exposure to lots of light helps to regulate the body's natural circadian rhythms, and sends a message that "This is day; this is when we're up." Then in the evening, especially on the long days of summer, start to close curtains and dim the house as a prep for the message "This is night; this is when we sleep."

- **Reserve the bedroom for sleep if you can**. This can be hard, since in many homes space is precious and the bedroom of the older adult with dementia is set up as a refuge for sitting, watching TV, and so on. But if you can spare the space, linking the room to sleep-only sometimes helps.

- **Follow "sleep hygiene" basics**: Keep the bedroom temperature on the cool side, with comfortable blankets for warmth as needed. It's best if it's dark, although most people need light to guide them to the bathroom. One solution is motion-sensor nightlights.

Tip: **"My wife is calmed by the humming sound of a fan. It's white noise that covers up street sounds. I run it even in winter, on low." —R.R.**

- **Consider a weighted blanket**. There's some evidence that it can help reduce anxiety, by encouraging relaxation, and this can help with sleep. The usual rule of thumb is to pick a blanket that's 10 percent of body weight plus another pound or two. If the person has respiratory or circulatory issues, check with a doctor or occupational therapist first.

- **Avoid laying out the next day's clothes at night when you're grappling with sleep issues**. Do it when the person wakes up to act as a visual cue to get up and get dressed.

- **During night wakings, avoid turning on bright lighting or the television**. Keep a consistent sense of difference between day and night.

- **Pay attention to caffeine consumption**. Many older adults have a big coffee habit. Caffeine doesn't just pep you up. It's a diuretic that makes you need to go to the bathroom. Try to wean your loved one off coffee and caffeinated tea after midday if sleep is becoming an issue.

- **Also beware of alcohol use, especially in the afternoon or evening**. A "nightcap" can make someone fall asleep but then awaken a short time later.

- **Avoid all "nighttime medicines** (with PM in the name) and antihistamines. These can worsen sleep.

- **Consider hiring night help, if you can afford it, to protect your own sleep**. If night wakings are chronic, an aide who works the overnight shift can help with toileting and getting back to sleep.

- **When behavioral strategies aren't working and your own health is in jeopardy, report persistent disrupted sleep to the doctor**. Seeing problems several times a week is a good rule of thumb. He or she can look for other underlying causes, such as depression. Have the doctor review all medications, also. In some cases, a referral to a sleep specialist can help (for a problem such as apnea, for example), but the person should have experience dealing with dementia (a geriatrician is best). What works for someone without dementia may not apply. Your doctor may explore sleep aids. Antipsychotic meds are used in some extreme cases, but they don't generally work for insomnia.

Tip: **"My husband had more sleep problems when he took Aricept in the evening. We switched it to the morning on the doctor's advice, and the problem really improved."** — **S.B.**

To help you cope:

- **Don't feel you need to stay up until the person falls back asleep if you're confident that she's safe**. Offer a quiet activity, such as a book on tape or playing the same classical music she listens to before going to bed. (TV is often too stimulating for many people, who mistake the scenes on the screen for real events and get worked up over them.) Some caregivers have had success using a baby monitor to keep tabs on a wakeful person in another room. It might provide enough sound contact to reassure you that she's okay and let you fall back asleep without getting out of bed.

- **Take sleep problems seriously**. Don't just "suck it up" and consider chronic sleep deprivation to be part of the bargain of Alzheimer's care. Occasional mixed-up days and some rough nights are one thing. But when the disruptions are chronic and extreme, spending the time and money to resolve the issue is critical. The health risks to you are just too great and too well documented.

It's absolutely worth it to bring in reinforcements: consulting a doctor, hiring night help. You may even want to hire an elder companion for an hour or so a day to give you time to nap.

- **Explore whether a change in care situations is the best solution**. When a sleep problem is really intractable (or in-home support isn't viable) it can be a message that it's time to explore an alternate care situation. Many families resist a move away from home, only to find that everyone's health improves afterwards (some nursing homes even have nighttime activities). That can also leave the caregiver better able to be an advocate, companion, and beloved figure to the person with Alzheimer's. Every case is different, but sleep really brings home the adage, never say never.

o o o

Sleeps Too Much

Some days, Su seemed fine. She'd sit around the house and watch TV, pet her cats, or "look at" the paper. But other days, she didn't want to get out of bed. If coaxed up, she'd fall asleep on the sofa after breakfast and sleep all day. She'd doze right through lunch and dinner. Her husband, Warren, first worried that all that sleep would keep her up at night, but she'd continue to sleep at night, too.

Then he worried about that. Is it possible to sleep too much?

WHY it happens:

Sleep is controlled deep in the brain. It's not surprising, then, that disrupted sleep patterns are a common effect of the brain erosion of Alzheimer's.

Stage of disease matters. Some people with mild-stage dementia report feeling excessively tired, possibly from working so hard to stay "with it" and "on" all day. Moderate dementia is when the more wakeful sleep problems typically pick up. Later in advanced Alzheimer's terminal stage, it's normal for the person to sleep more and more as a natural part of the dying process as the body is slowly shutting down.

Other possible causes (or additional causes):

- *An underlying physical problem, such as an infection.* Excessive lethargy can be a warning sign of delirium.

- *A medication interaction* or side effect.

- *Depression.* Disordered sleep is one of the key warning signs.

While sleeping too little or too erratically tends to cause more problems for caregivers, sleeping too much can also be problematic. The lack of a consistent schedule can, over time, make someone cranky and cause other behavior problems to increase. Or, over time, the person's day and night schedule can flip-flop.

In general, people think and feel better and have more energy when sleep is regular. Excessive daytime sleep can lead to disturbed behavior in the evening.

TRY this:

- **Mention excessive sleep to the doctor**, especially if it's a recent change or if you're seeing behavioral and mood changes, too. You want to make sure there isn't some other problem or medication causing sleep changes.

- **For someone who's fairly "with it" when awake, make sure that she gets regular exercise and time outdoors**. Too much sleep can make people drowsy, but movement peps them up and makes them more likely to sleep normally.

- **Don't over-worry**. Of all the challenges in dementia care, this one actually makes life a bit easier on families, assuming the excessive sleep is not disruptive.

o o o

Walking Trouble, Shuffling

One of the more distressing physical changes in my dad was the way he walked. Even deep in his retirement, through his 70s, he'd traipse a half mile to buy the daily newspaper rather than get home delivery. He resisted a golf cart longer than many of his buddies. But as his dementia took hold, he became more frail.

Going anywhere was an excruciating lesson in patience, as he slooooooowly maneuvered out of the car and began to walk. He was still mobile through the end of his life, but he seemed to have trouble picking up his feet and moving them along.

I didn't learn until later that he was doing the "Alzheimer's shuffle," a common kind of impaired gait. —P.S.S.

WHY it happens:

A shuffling walk reflects the difficulty that the brain and body are having communicating. As the parietal lobe part of the brain, which governs motor skills, is affected, so is muscle coordination. The affected person has trouble picking up his feet to walk and drags them a bit. You may also notice that he's unsteady and begins to stoop. Sometimes you see him concentrating harder on each step.

Although families don't often pick up on a slowing gait until the middle stage of Alzheimer's, some research indicates changes in walking may actually be one of the earlier symptoms. Gait changes can be seen even before memory changes. Problems with walking are strongly associated with vascular dementia, too.

Movement involves the nervous system (sending messages throughout the body) as well as the heart and muscles. Some studies have revealed that people with cognitive impairment show more pronounced trouble walking when asked to do a thinking-skill task at the same time. As they divert focus to the cognitive task, their walking worsens. Slowing walking speed is also associated with more cognitive decline.

A shuffle can be worsened by a fear of falling, due to changes in depth perception or orientation caused by dementia. The apprehension makes the person take more tentative steps. Ironically, fear of falling is one of the risk factors for falling more.

A reaction to medication and other chronic diseases that add to overall frailty can also contribute to shaky walking. Medications that worsen balance include anticholinergics (found in overactive bladder drugs, PM painkillers, and some antidepressants), sedatives, some blood pressure meds, and opiate painkillers.

Falls are the real danger here. A quarter of those who fall and break a hip die within six months, and half can't return to a private home and relocate to a nursing facility.

Someone with vision problems, whether related to Alzheimer's or a pre-existing condition, is at added danger of falling.

TRY this:

- **Make sure shoes fit well**. Look for soles that offer some traction, neither too slick nor too rigid, such as canvas sneakers or sport sandals with secure back straps. Beware sport shoes with super-thick treads. These can actually contribute to falls because they can stick to the carpet if the wearer can't easily lift his foot. While laces are ideal for a snug fit, they can come undone and be tripping hazards. They're also hard to tie for someone with poor flexibility and muscle-control issues. Stick with Velcro straps. Pay attention to size. Nine in ten women wear shoes that are too small, says the American Association of Orthopedic Surgeons. Older adults tend to go by the size they've "always been" or don't realize how easy it now is to find wide-width shoes.

- **Don't overlook safe slippers, since people with dementia often move around a lot at night**. Slippers should have treads, too, and fasten securely to feet. Avoid scuff-style footwear and flip-flops.

- **Consider encouraging bare feet indoors**. An Irish study in the journal *Age and Ageing* reported that frail older women who wore shoes fell more than those who went barefoot.

- **Provide a cane, walking stick, or walker to boost support and, in turn, confidence**. Of the three, walkers carry the lowest risk of falling, but they're often met with more resistance at first. Many people resist them because it makes them feel "old." Emphasize the advantages of a walking device: You'll be able to walk better or farther, exercise will help you grow stronger, and you'll be less likely to fall and break a bone, which will really make you feel old.

- **When walking in stores, encourage the person to push a shopping cart**. It can provide just the right added support.

- **Offer constant reminders to use the assistive device, since the person will likely forget**. Store it in view as a visual reminder.

- **De-clutter**. Lower the risk of accidental trips by getting rid of throw rugs, piles of paper, loose electric cords, and any other objects that encumber pathways. Pet toys are a surprisingly common source of danger.

- **Beware of two-toned rugs or other places where there's a contrast in floor color on one level**. This can be perceived as a step, causing the person to jerk the leg up on a level surface. The best floor coverings for someone with walking and perception problems: monotone, low-pile, wall-to-wall carpeting that extends seamlessly into hallways and other rooms.

- **Offer extra support on steps and curbs**. Changes in depth perception can make it easy to misjudge these distances, putting someone with dementia off balance.

Tip: "**I painted the steps from the house down to the garage in alternating colors, red and white. Before, the concrete made them all look the same. The stripes are funky, but the contrast really helps my mother, and it helps me, too! —J.R.**

- **Mention any trouble walking to the doctor at the next checkup**, especially if it's a recent change or there's been a change in medications. It's always smart to rule out or treat other causes.

- **Ask about a referral to a physical therapist or occupational therapist**. These experts won't be able to make the dementia shuffle go away, but they can evaluate balance and gait, and offer advice on how to best reduce the risk of falls, including showing how to use a walking assistive device.

- **Check vision**. Make sure prescriptions are up-to-date and glasses lenses are clean.

- **Do what you can to keep your loved one moving**, even if it's slow. Regular movement can reduce the risk of falls.

- **Resist the urge to try to hurry the person along with your words**. Saying, "Hurry!" Or, "We'll be late!" only adds stress and can tank your progress.

To help you cope:

- **Allow more time to get places**. You'll feel less maddened with impatience if you get in the habit of building in time for the slowed pace.

- **Go a little Zen**. Take deep breaths and remind yourself that all that matters is this moment, and this next step, and the next.

o o o

"Alzheimer's is a family disease."
—Carol Burnett, actress and comic

4: HELP FOR PERSONAL AND FAMILY STRESSORS

When "everything else" undermines you

At one point, my brother Paul and sister-in-law Laura had three parents living with them. Only one had dementia (my dad). But the entire trio was north of age 75, and the myriad health issues between them—cancer, congestive heart failure, vertigo, to name a few—made for plenty of doctor visits, medicines to track, and symptoms to watch. Oh, and this cozy, crazy abode also housed six kids under age 13, three cats, and two dogs. (Luckily, my brother's a builder and kept remodeling his house accordingly.)

Not surprisingly, my sister-in-law, a.k.a. The Saint, soon developed terrible insomnia. She often couldn't eat. Some days, despite her mile-long to-do list, she couldn't get out of bed. Finally one night, her symptoms landed her in the E.R.

Diagnosis: physically healthy but emotionally and mentally exhausted.

As part of her long road to learning to take care of herself as well as she took care of everyone else, we struck a deal: Whenever she was feeling frayed, she was to call me, at any hour. And whenever she and my brother were truly unraveling, I'd come to provide some respite care. Never have I contributed a relatively small amount of time in a way that made such a huge difference.

You can't provide dementia care without an escape hatch or two— or ten. I've included this section because although direct-care skills are critical, families also need tools to battle the other dragons that affect their lives as caregivers: pesky people, work-life conflicts, too little time, and our own good intentions.

o o o

STRESS—AND WHAT FEEDS IT

The stress of dementia care is so real you can touch it—in your aching head, tense shoulders, sore back, sick stomach, clenched jaw.

Goodness knows it's touching you. Study after survey shows that caregivers report more stress than non-caregivers. One report from the American Psychological Association named caregivers as one of the three most stressed groups in the land, along with the depressed and the obese. Many who provide long-term Alzheimer's care wear this Triple Crown.

Fully 90 percent of Alzheimer's caregivers say that emotional stress is their number-one challenge, a 2017 survey found.

Stress devastates your body and your mind. Much as I love health statistics, I'm not going to further raise your blood pressure and risk of depression by reciting all the perils here. You already know that everything from your weight and mental state to your heart health and immune system are put at risk when you assume the care of another human being with dementia. Caregivers are twice as likely to smoke and 25 percent more likely to binge drink.

Stress also leads to burnout. Professionals call it "compassion fatigue"—caring so much that you give yourself too little. "Stress is all about 'too much' – too much work, too much activity, too much stimulus. Burnout is 'too little' – too little time, too little interest, too little energy," says Patricia Smith, a certified compassion fatigue specialist in Mountain View, California, and founder of the Compassion Fatigue Awareness Project.

When you're stressed, the cause may seem obvious: a big medical bill, a fight with your spouse over parent care, a health scare, or all of the above. Yet the real stressor—the thing that sends the heart racing and the head pounding is often the way we react to a given situation. This doesn't mean that just thinking differently will wipe out credit card debt or make a sick person better. But it means that your mental and practical responses can make or break how well you weather the storm.

As you face a given stress factor, think about what might be really feeding your anxiety and tension. Realizing that there's often both an immediate problem and a less obvious one can help you move toward a solution that's more constructive than alcohol, comfort food, a day under the covers, or worse.

These are five such "hidden" causes of stress for caregivers:

Underlying stressor #1: Lack of control

You sense: "I feel stuck." "I don't have any good options." "Nobody asks what I think." "It's hopeless."

What helps: Find ways you can exert influence, even if they're small ones like gathering information. When our action-oriented brains feel like we're making progress, we feel more in control.

Ask yourself:

- Can I do anything to change the situation? Or am I stuck out of habit?

- Have I turned over every stone?

- Am I asking for more help or authority? Can I assert myself more?

- Have I given up too easily? Who else could I talk to? Have I called the local Area Agency on Aging to find out about local resources that might be able to help?

- Have I asked my human resources office at work about resources?

- Am I moving toward a better situation because of small changes I'm making, even if it's tough now?

Underlying stressor #2: Unrealistic expectations or standards

You sense: "Nobody can [fill in the blank] the way I do." "I'm the only one who gets it." "I should be able to manage better." "I'm always disappointed by the way they...."

What helps: Take stock of where your notions about how things "should" be or how people (including yourself) "ought" to behave came from. Much as we'd all like to be perfect, nobody—not even Mother Teresa, if you'd asked her—ever reached that lofty point.

Ask yourself:

- Am I truly being reasonable here, given the constraints of time, money, and the way this disease works?

- Am I defining success and progress realistically? Who could give me a reality check?

- Why do I think something must happen a certain way?

- What would happen if it unfolded differently?

- What's the worst that could happen?

- What can I move off my to-do list by delegating, hiring help, or crossing out (spotless windows, I'm talking to you!)?

Underlying stressor #3: Uncertainty or fear

You sense: "I don't know what to expect." "How will we manage?" "What fresh hell awaits today?" "I'm terrified that things will get worse."

What helps: That old cliché "knowledge is power" also happens to be darn good advice. Reality is often frightening, to be sure. But the more you know, the more informed your perspective, and that can tamp down some of the runaway anxiety that can intensify fear.

Ask yourself:

- Have I collected enough facts from reliable sources?

- Have I made lists of questions for the doctor so I don't miss anything at appointments?

- Have I talked to other people about dementia caregiving? Whatever your situation, you're not the first person who's gone through it.

- Have I started making what-if plans, so that I'll be better prepared at the next juncture? Things that help include arranging the appropriate legal, financial, and advanced-care paperwork, looking into home modifications (say, for a wheelchair) or home-care aides, and exploring housing options.

- Am I maybe looking for answers to questions that can't be answered?

- Am I worrying about what's real today and tomorrow, or getting way ahead of myself?

Underlying stressor #4: Too little self-respect

You sense: "I don't have time for myself." "With all I put up with, I deserve this pint of ice cream." "If I were stronger/more organized/more attentive, I wouldn't be so stressed out." "I hate myself."

What helps: Start by loving yourself even more than all the other people you love. That can be a tall order for the generous personality type that's often attracted to caregiving. Some caregivers suffer from "big-hearted disease," always thinking about others first. Carers need advocates, too—ourselves.

Ask yourself:

- Am I good to myself? Or am I "rewarding" myself in ways that make me feel better in the moment but will make me feel much worse in a few hours? (That's the story of a bag of potato chips or a bottle of booze.)

- Am I even on my daily priority list? Or have I allowed myself to be crowded out by everyone else?

- Do I feel likeable and deserving of love? (Everyone is! But if you have trouble seeing yourself this way, it's time to find a counselor who can help you unlock this block.)

- What am I going to do for some "me" time today?

- When is the last time I had a physical exam? Do I know what my blood pressure, cholesterol levels, and other markers are saying about my own health —and am I figuring out even small ways I can improve them?

- How can I arrange a short getaway? Who could help me, and what do I need to do to make it happen?

Underlying stressor #5: Feeling isolated or unsupported

You sense: "Nobody understands." "They call to ask about [my mother/my father/my spouse], but never about me." "I'm too embarrassed (or depressed, or overwhelmed) to socialize."

What helps: Force yourself to reach out—even if it's not your natural tendency and even if it feels like another task on your to-do list. Social and emotional isolation fuel a creeping despair that nips at all caregivers. Brainstorm every opportunity to break out of its grasp by connecting with others. That includes in person, online, by phone, via community resources, via hired help, every stone you can overturn. Some of us have greater social needs than others, but every dementia caregiver needs some degree of connection with the outside world.

Ask yourself:

- Have I spoken out to anyone about how I feel or what help I need? Who?

- Am I actively seeking help, or have I been content just to grouse?

- Who's in my personal care circle? Who can I turn to for emotional support as well as for practical help? This is a new life situation and calls for a fresh support network of those who have either been there or truly get it. A few sessions with a counselor or therapist are covered by most insurance plans and can make all the difference.

- Have I called a friend or talked to one online today?

- When was the last time I got out of the house—and how can I do it again tomorrow? Look into respite programs, day programs, and elder companions for your loved one, so you can circulate in the world a bit.

Finally, these insights from the super-stressed:

At the Duke Center for Aging Alzheimer's Family Support Program in Durham, N.C., social worker Bobbi Matchar has led an eight-week memory loss education and support group called Memory Makers since 2012, and a spin-off friendship group for "graduates" called the Alpha Community. What helps fuel resilience for the participating care partners? They say it's the following stress-reducing nuggets, as reported by Matchar and program director Lisa Gwyther at the 2017 World Congress of Geriatrics and Gerontology:

Celebrate small victories: "It ain't fun, it stinks, it sucks sometimes. But we can still have a few good moments."

Rely on humor: "Sometimes there are totally absurd things you can't control and you just have to laugh."

Take a good-enough approach: "If a family member with dementia wears two different shoes...so what?"

Accept what can't be controlled: "There's no such thing as 'hurry up' in our house."

Be flexible and creative: One woman told her husband the newly hired companion was a fitness trainer.

Hang onto the love: Many said they showed signs of affection even when it didn't match their feelings.

Give yourself credit for your strengths: "I didn't think I could do this," many said. But they did.

o o o

FAMILY-RELATED STRESSORS

Absence of Family Help

Some common scenarios:

All talk, no action: "Let me know if I can help!" says the relative. But when you ask, the would-be helper is inevitably busy that day. Or worse, she cancels at the last minute. Her life always takes priority over yours.

Out of sight, out of mind: Family members who aren't on the scene seem to simply vanish. They might call and ask how the person with Alzheimer's is doing, in a perfunctory way, but they never bother to ask how you're holding up. Or they just assume you have things covered and vamoose.

Not my thing: Some people have really creative reasons for not being able to help: "It makes me sad to see him this way." "I'm just not very good around old people." "It would be too depressing/too stressful/too upsetting for me." "I'm not in the best of health myself you know; I have migraines." "I'd rather remember him the way he used to be." (Yes, these are all real excuses family caregivers have reported hearing.)

What you should know about lack of help:

The bottom line: People either want to help or they don't.

Often people want to lend a hand but hang back for legitimate reasons. They may not be sure how to offer their assistance or what kind would make a difference. When they offer, a caregiver may fall into that social-niceness dance of shrugging it off, and then the helper doesn't persist. Some people do feel awkward around older adults or those with Alzheimer's—even close family members—and can benefit from a little hand-holding and education. It can also help to invite them to handle tasks or responsibilities that may be less hands-on but just as beneficial to you. Ironically, some caregivers make their tasks look so easy (and complain so little) that family members don't even suspect they're needed.

If there's one truism about help when caring for someone with Alzheimer's, it's that more is always better.

Sadly, some people truly don't want to help. It may have to do with their own internal conflicts, problems, or feelings about the person with Alzheimer's, or it could have to do with their relationship with

285

you. You may never know.

What can help you:

- **Make lists!** Write down everything you must do to run your life and manage care. When someone asks how he or she can help, whip out the list and ask back, "Great, how about X or Y?"

- **Get a firm commitment**. Well-intentioned helpers are more likely to follow through when you get them to specify dates and times. Open your calendar in front of them. Then record the help offer on both your calendars—and send reminders if you have to.

- **Set up repeat gigs**. Your nephew driving your mom to a hair appointment is great. Having him do it every month? Way better.

- **Remember that "help" has many definitions**. It can take the form of hands-on care, time, transportation, escape, paperwork, research, financial support, moral support, or caregiving relief. Because I'm self-employed, for example, it was easy for me to be back-up caregiver for my dad during the time he lived with my brother a couple of hours away. In between, I made a point of calling my sister-in-law often just to be a sounding board and source of stress release. She also knew she could call me at any hour (and did!). It was a small thing on my part, but sometimes the difference between going bonkers and holding on another day is a small thing.

- **Don't waste precious time and emotional energy beating your head against a wall**. If family members rebuff you repeatedly, give up. Yes, I said give up. Sometimes you have to "accept what you cannot change" and let go of the resentment, anger, and frustration that builds up when those who ought to step up instead choose to step back. Your emotional energy is valuable. Spend it on making life better for the person with dementia—and yourself—in the ways that are in your control.

- **Look outside the family circle**. When family won't help, redouble your efforts to tap into community resources that can, starting with the clearinghouse Area Agency on Aging.

- **Shore up personal support for yourself.** A support group can offer hive-mind problem solving and idea sharing, along with opportunities to vent a little, which caregivers forced into lone-soldier syndrome especially need.

- **Be sure you're not part of the problem.** Some caregivers wind up as Lone Rangers because that's exactly how they set things up. They fail to reach out to others when it's needed. Or they rebuff help that's offered. They don't want to "bother" anyone. They make excuses. Let go of old ideas that asking for help is a sign of weakness. If ever you needed other people in your life, it's now.

Caregivers may also fall into the rut of believing that nobody can do it as well as they can. Gail Sheehy, author of *Passages in Caregiving*, calls this "playing God." She says she felt personally responsible for warding off all disasters and dangers while caring for her husband. While it's true in many cases that the hands-on caregiver does the best job, many others can do a good job. A nobody-can-do-it-like-me attitude ultimately doesn't add up to the common good. You need help. Most people are willing to help. The person with dementia will manage just fine under someone else's temporary watch and may in fact enjoy new faces and a break from 24/7 you.

o o o

A Family Favorite

Some common scenarios:

The swoop-in, swoop-out superhero: Sibling A lives near her parents and is there day-in, day-out helping with everything from doctor appointments to medication reminders. She feels taken for granted. Sibling B lives across the country—swoops in twice a year to visit and dazzles the parents with her attention and care. Never mind that she then disappears after stirring up half-baked plans and hopes, seldom to be heard from until the next hero's welcome.

The halo effect: Sometimes one sibling Can Do No Wrong and the other...well, Is Never Right. Often a parent will defer to the eldest, or to a son over a daughter, or to the child who lives closest.

Old wounds: A perceived rivalry can be rooted in decades-old competitive feelings...he always let you get away with things...she gets more because she's the baby...Dad never took me seriously....

Sibling Olympics: Some hyper-competitive siblings strive to out-care one another. They duke it out for recognition as Most Dutiful Daughter, undermining one another's efforts along the way. Mom or Dad agrees with whomever they last talked to. Although it's much more common to have too few devoted caregivers, rather than too many, any situation where everyone's not on the same page can be dangerous.

What you should know about favoritism:

Can you say infuriating? Of course you can if you feel that you're a bypassed sibling.

The favoritism may be real or only seem that way. Perception is a big part of the problem. But parents do show preferences. Research has recently debunked the idealized notion that mothers don't have favorites. Purdue's J. Jill Suitor and Cornell's Karl Pillemer, both sociologists, did a series of studies with hundreds of women ages 65 to 75. Most admitted feeling emotionally closest to daughters (four times more often than sons) and youngest children. In a crisis, though, they'd turn to a firstborn for advice. Perceived favoritism ripples all through life, say Suitor and Pillemer. Those who sensed it growing up tend to grapple more with depression as adults.

Here's the really interesting part: When the women were re-interviewed at 72 and 82, the child they'd felt closest to wound up playing caregiver three-quarters of the time. But when a different child fell into that role, the mothers were more often depressed. Research published by Pillemer in 2013 shows that the preferred child tends to share values with the mother, live nearby, and yes, be a daughter.

To some degree, it's a like-it-or-lump-it situation, because you can't change your parents' feelings or how you feel about them. The difficulty is that these perceptions can get in the way of both giving good care and protecting your own health and sense of self-worth.

The going can get roughest when it seems like there's disparity over:

- *Finances.* Who "gets" more or is being dealt a fair hand gets tangled in the roots of childhood rivalry, which is a craving for equal love and attention from parents. And, very sad to say, some people get greedy as a relative grows more infirm.

- *Legal influence.* Fears over who's exacting the most control over health care decisions or legal-financial decisions get dicey, because powers of attorney are often held by one person, rather than shared.

- *An uneven burden of care.* It's bad enough to do the lion's share of work. It's harder when you feel like someone who does less is rewarded more.

The dynamics can get trickier when adult siblings don't even know one another very well. It's not uncommon for kids to grow up, move away, and have few day-to-day dealings with one another. They may never develop adult relationships. They're stuck in old childhood ways of interacting (often featuring lots of immature competition and bickering). Parents, too, may not have strong or realistic adult-to-adult relationships with grown children. They may fall into old patterns that serve neither party well. Then, when a crisis hits that requires everyone to pull together and communicate, everyone's ill-equipped to do so.

What can help you:

- **Be sure you're assessing a situation realistically**. Are your hackles up because of what's being done (or not done) or because you're reacting to some personality trait or pattern in a sibling? You may well be in the right, but it's important to separate past grudges from what's best in the present situation.

- **Talk about your roles in concrete ways**. "Rivalries re-emerge because we no longer know who is who in our family, or at least, who does what," notes Francine Russo in *They're Your Parents, Too*, her guide to sibling relationships in eldercare. It can help to step back from your assumptions. Talk together about how weird this dynamic is. Say, okay, who's going to gather which information? How are we going to make decisions? What do we do when we can't agree?

- **Focus on the big picture**. It's common, and easy, to resent someone who comes in from afar to stir things up and give glamorous input when you're the one who does the dirty work day-in, day-out. Try not to take it personally that their relatively small efforts are applauded while yours go unrecognized, and just let it go in the interest of the big picture. (Yes, it's especially rankling when the hero-for-a-day doesn't acknowledge all you do.)

- **Try bringing in outside help**. If everyone agrees, try meeting with a geriatric care manager or an eldercare mediator (a family mediator with expertise in aging issues). These impartial experts are skilled at cutting through the layers of family squabbles. Try using the argument that you're all in this for the long haul (the rest of your lives), and a neutral third-party can both do what's best for the person with dementia and preserve your future relationships.

o o o

Criticism

Some common scenarios:

Endless second-guessing: One sibling is the primary caregiver. She's doing 99 percent of the work AND doing her best to keep the others informed. But instead of getting a sympathetic ear or any kind of help, they question her every decision: "Why this medication and not that one?" "I've heard a better thing to do is...." "That lawyer is a crook; you should have used a different one."

Sharing problems but no solutions: Some people like to point out what's wrong without offering a better way. Nutrition, socialization, hygiene, finances—any topic of care is fair game. Often, of course, the hands-on caregiver is well aware of a problem or a situation that's less than ideal (mom hates getting a bath, the local day program is too expensive). We want help, not a restatement of the obvious.

Laying blame: Some people need a demon. Rather than blaming the disease for taking away a loved one, they project their distress on the primary caregiver. Situations that are nobody's 'fault" get unfairly pinned on that person: "You let him wander away—where were you?" "She's in the hospital again?" "How did she get these bedsores?"

What you should know about criticism:

Fault-finders often operate on auto-pilot. It's their reflexive way of seeing the world. And when they're feeling guilty or insecure, it's as if they go on a finger-pointing mission. Unconsciously, they're asking themselves, *How can I make you feel bad so I feel better?* Judgmental people tend to pick on the handiest scapegoat they can find. The perfect target: a relative or friend whom they perceive as being closer to the person with Alzheimer's, or doing more, or knowing more.

Devaluing someone else through shame or blame makes a critic feel superior (even if their accusations aren't true), relieving their insecurity, guilt, or low self-esteem—at least temporarily.

Criticism isn't always a psychological power play, of course. The critic may intend to be helpful, not hurtful, or may just be saying things in a clumsy way. Maybe she's a Type A personality who sees something that needs fixing and can't help herself, for example. Sometimes criticisms are made off-the-cuff, the thoughtless comments or uninformed questions of someone who sees the dementia only in small doses and doesn't have a real sense of what you're going through. Before you get your hackles up, consider whether the critic "gets" what's going on.

And, of course, if the criticisms are coming from the person with dementia, you have to factor this in to your response. Hearing such digs is every bit as deflating as when they come from someone else, but the origin is different. Here, the root of criticism and complaints is usually disease-triggered fear or insecurity.

What can help you:

- **Use "criticism IQ."** First, use "I" statements that play back how the hurtful words make you feel: "I feel hurt when you talk to me like that." "I really feel upset when you criticize every decision I make." "I feel uncomfortable around you because I never know when your criticisms are coming or why you make them." When you say you're hurt by a critic's words, it takes away the emotional distance that makes it easier to keep on criticizing. Then the "Q" part. With a question, invite the critic to suggest a specific approach or improvement he or she is willing to handle or collaborate on: "Why don't you be in charge of X?" "Tell me what you'd be willing to do instead and how." And follow up: "Will you make that happen? How? When?"

- **Sidestep getting roped into further judgments on your character**. Bullies often respond with comments like, "Oh, you're too sensitive!" "I'm only trying to help if you'd let me!" It's a way of masking their pushiness by turning it back on you. Say, "I can't help my reaction." "I'd like your help, but your tone is hurtful and unproductive."

- **Don't argue**. You only give a fault-finder an excuse to justify the criticism and belittle you further. You're much more empowered if you can turn the discussion away from the critic's perceptions of you to your own feelings—and a collaborative effort toward a solution.

- **Turn their words back on them**. Without arguing, try to move the conversation in a more constructive direction: "What can you do to change that?" "That's an interesting opinion. Tell me what you'd do differently and how." (These tips don't always work with a really toxic critic, so if you're not hearing true help, abandon this strategy.)

- **Don't let yourself believe unfounded criticisms**. A criticism carries two parts—the perceived fault ("You let Dad wander off!") and the hidden meaning implied ("therefore you're a jerk!"). Once you realize this, you can see why some criticism really stings. "But if you choose not to buy into the 'that makes me bad,' part, you're inoculated against the dart; it's not going to hurt you," says Pepperdine University psychotherapist Steve Sultanoff.

- **Don't apologize automatically if you're not in the wrong**. ("Oh, sorry, sorry!") That doesn't smooth things over. It only feeds bullying behavior. Better: Delete the word "sorry" and stand up for yourself.

- **Decide whether the criticisms seem to stem from really knowing the situation**. If so, invite the critic to spend more time with the person who has dementia, such as subbing for you while you run errands or taking over weekend care. There's nothing like hands-on experience to make someone see a situation differently.

- **Applaud yourself and all you do**. Describing yourself in a negative light ("I'm boring," "I'm bad at talking to doctors") is just piling on. Pep talk that's positive, on the other hand, might feel corny ("That was a nice reply!" "Good hair day!") but has been shown to actually make us feel better. If you're constantly being taken down by others, take a few minutes each day to talk yourself up.

- **Keep your distance**. Ultimately, your health comes first. You're well within your rights to avoid those who only want to level you, especially if they do nothing in the way of balancing their snipes with practical, emotional, or financial support.

- **Listen for a nugget of truth**. Criticism isn't always unfounded or unwarranted. Try to listen neutrally, with an open mind, to see if there's anything eye-opening or useful you can pluck from what at first sounds like an attack. After all, people have different values, life experiences, contacts, and other influences on how they react to situations. Ask yourself what a critic might be seeing through the lens of their experience to make them say what they did. A sibling who lives far away may sense a parent's decline more quickly that someone who sees them every day, for example. Or someone with medical expertise can have helpful knowledge to share, even if they express it less than gracefully.

o o o

Denial

Some common scenarios:

Problem, what problem? After my mom fell and broke her pelvis, and the degree of my dad's worsening dementia became obvious, my siblings and I began to discuss their living situation after the immediate crisis ended. To some of the five us, it seemed obvious that their days of living independently without any kind of help were numbered. But some siblings weren't convinced. They said things like, "This is just a short-term problem...Let's not get ahead of ourselves... Dad's just getting older...."

Making excuses: Some people would rather blame anything other than Alzheimer's for what's going on: age, recovery from surgery, orneriness, disorientation from a move, etc. There may be a few grains of truth in there. Unfortunately, such an attitude gets in the way of getting everyone on board to do things like protect finances, curb dangerous driving, start medications or other therapies, and so on.

Too close for discomfort: The person who's nearest to the one with cognitive trouble—a spouse, the adult child who lives next-door—sometimes has more denial than more distant family. Those who are farther away often have the advantage of noticing changes more immediately. To someone who's there every day, incremental changes can be less visible.

Self-denial: It's not uncommon for caregivers to have an unrealistic sense of the situation they're in. They think they can do it alone, for example, or put up with situations long after they're unsafe. Those with a large capacity for suffering beyond what many healthy people would consider tolerable can cling to a warped perception of reality for a long time.

Denial by owner: The person in denial is often the person with dementia. Early in the disease, when awareness is still intact, the person may refuse to admit anything's amiss—or just refuse to talk about it.

What you should know about denial:

Denial—refusing to face facts—is usually rooted in fear. Someone in denial may be afraid of what's ahead, known or unknown. Like the proverbial ostrich with its head in the sand, it becomes easier not to see a problem than to face it.

For some, the stakes are too high to face reality. They have too much vested in their own illusion of the way things are now. ("I'm busy in my career. I'm sure Dad and Mom are fine on their own." "I still feel like a kid myself. Dad can't be losing it yet!") That version of reality might not be logical, but they cling to it.

Another contributing factor: Alzheimer's can be so startling and strange that we're willing to consider any other explanation for what's going on, no matter how implausible. Some people will even turn the issue into a fault of yours ("Why are you looking for trouble?") rather than see a situation that needs addressing. The stigma around dementia can be intimidating or paralyzing.

It may feel easier to be in denial (for a while), but the dangers are multifold:

- *Denial can get in the way of getting good care or making a situation safer.* Many families make excuses ("It's not that bad...") until the person is lost on the highway, having driven across three state lines.

- *Denial can make everyday life harder.* If you don't see a situation realistically, you're less likely to get sufficient help. You might hold onto expectations for how your loved one should behave and wind up chronically disappointed or exhausted.

- *Denial can strain relationships.* When one person isn't even seeing the problem, it's hard to strategize together about a solution.

- *Denial can interfere with quality of life.* This is often seen at the end of life, when families are resistant to discuss hospice or palliative care because they're in denial about the specter of death. Instead of a peaceful last chapter, there may be intrusive hospitalizations and family disagreement.

It's important to realize that although people who are sick are often in denial about their own condition, Alzheimer's presents a different type of denial. Someone with Alzheimer's eventually lacks the capacity to understand what's going on in his own brain. This kind of denial, more like obliviousness, is especially challenging for families, because it requires a different set of skills to deal with it.

What can help you:

- **Give a denier a little space**. Denial can be a shock absorber for the soul, a coping mechanism that allows people to maintain sanity and get used to a change. Some people need more time than others to face the realities of a difficult situation.

- **Decide how much someone else's denial is a problem for you**. Some denial gets in the way of help. Other times it's just vexing because it means others don't agree with you—but it doesn't really affect your day-to-day life.

- **Separate denial from lack of knowledge**. Denial is refusing to acknowledge facts—but you have to have the facts in the first place. Be sure that the person having a hard time accepting a situation at least understands the options, symptoms, treatments, or other relevant information. Present the full story, with a written record of worrisome incidents. Share informative books or articles. Encourage conversations with doctors, other experts, or friends who have been in similar situations.

- **Record visual proof**. Seeing is believing. Make a video of your dad limping: "See how hard it is for him to walk?" It can be especially persuasive if you can compare it to an earlier recording. Or tape a conversation with your mom showing her confusion that you can play later for siblings: "See? I'm not making this up!"

- **Avoid lording your take on the situation over someone who's in denial**. If you're confident of the truth, take comfort in that and keep your ego out of the dispute. It's about what to do, not who got there first.

- **Encourage talk about the very thing that's being avoided**. Ask gently: "Why do you think Mom will be able to live alone in this two-story house when the doctor said she won't be able to walk again?" "What do you think is the reason Dad keeps repeating himself and getting lost?"

- **Probe with hypotheticals**: It's easier for some people to imagine "pretend" situations rather than the ones they currently see. "What if Mom's mistakes with driving continue; what will happen? How will you feel if she gets hurt or hurts someone?" "What would be the worst that would happen if we talked to someone from hospice, just to learn more about it?" These scenarios can nudge the person along in his or her thinking.

- **Don't confuse denial with giving up hope**. Having hope means you're moving forward based on a clear grasp of reality: the dire and the unknowable, maybe seasoned with faith. Hope is a commodity that most people feel is a help, not a hindrance, and one you needn't abandon in any situation. Denial, in contrast, means avoiding reality because it's too painful to behold, which usually also means denying help (such as stronger pain meds, more adult day care, the comfort of assisted living, or palliative care).

o o o

Disagreement

Some common scenarios:

How to pay for care and other financial matters: Money matters are a top source of friction. One sibling wants to sell the family home. The other feels everything possible should be done to keep Mom in familiar surroundings. A well-to-do sibling expects the others to contribute an equal share. Spouses disagree over the terms of a will.

Medical conundrums: To operate or not to operate? This medication or that one? Participate in a clinical trial or no? When the patient in question can't reliably make his own decisions, families may not agree on what he'd prefer or what's in his best interest. Often there isn't one "right" answer.

Mom always liked you best! Disagreements can have deep roots. When our birth families are involved, we often revert back to childhood roles, and with them, the slights and perceptions that were formed during those years. Charges of favoritism can cause arguments. So can birth order's built-in expectations, such as the eldest expecting the younger sibs to go along with him, or that the youngest has no idea what she's talking about.

It's not your business! A wife dealing with her husband's memory problems might not like what her daughter has to say about the matter. A live-in caregiver feels she has a different perspective from her sister who lives 100 miles away. A stepson's opinion is valued less than a son's, even though the two were practically raised together.

What you should know about disagreement:

All families argue. Whether your relations over the years have been generally harmonious or always cantankerous, you can count on the fact that dealing with Alzheimer's is going to create friction. If you've always had problems, they're apt to intensify. If you've never had discord before, get ready.

That's partly because you're in a situation where emotions run high. Many decisions, large and small, must be made about the person's care, living situation, independence, medical condition, and that ultra-hot topic (whether Alzheimer's is present or not), money. Everyone involved has his or her own values, life experiences, and unique relationship with the person affected. You may be as close as can be with Dad, but your stepmother, your husband, and your daughter each have their own very personal connection. The same facts can look surprisingly different from each vantage point.

The trick is to manage discord before it eats away at you or your relationships and gets in the way of care.

Arguments are often fed by some of the other stressors discussed in this chapter: resentment, depression, and favoritism, for example.

What can help you:

- **Agree to disagree**. First, realize that there are some issues where everyone won't be on board, and that's okay. Separate the small stuff from the biggies.

- **Keep everyone in the loop as best you can**. Sometimes people quibble because they're not up to date on the facts or they're actually objecting to being left out. For some families, family meetings (possibly including the person with dementia) serve this purpose. Other ways to do this include conference calls or video chats, email updates, private group chats, private Facebook pages, or online care-circle services. Keeping written records of expenditures, health matters, and resources used puts things in black and white, which can help insulate you in the event of later attacks.

- **Keep the focus squarely on the person in need**. Relationships are complex. Emotions run high. Ask yourself if you're locked in a showdown whether it's really about the problem being discussed or about conflicting personalities. Sometimes what can seem like a disagreement over how to proceed is really a reactionary push-me-pull-you tug-of-war in which one party just can't stand for the other one to be right. Remind siblings or adult children: "This is about Mom; it's not about me or you."

- **Ask, "What do you think?"** Try stepping back from pushing your point of view and ask for advice. Even if you think the advice is wrong, just listen. This approach can disarm someone who wants to tangle. It often breaks the fight dynamic, allowing you to move to a more collaborative plane.

- **Divide and conquer**. You don't have to all agree or contribute in equal measure about everything. In many families, members have different domains of expertise. Among my own siblings, for example, a sister in the insurance business managed the paperwork. A builder brother handled household repairs and modifications. I held the medical power of attorney and took care of interactions with doctors. My older sister and sister-in-law excelled at moral support and hands-on care. We compared notes on the big stuff but mostly let each person make smaller decisions within his or her area of expertise. This approach has the added advantage of lightening the workload, so it doesn't all fall on one person. (My mom, an only child, used to say that the silver lining in caring for her mother's long decline with Alzheimer's was that at least she didn't have to argue with anybody else about her decisions.)

- **Solicit advice from neutral others**. Try asking strangers in chat groups or friends if they've had a similar situation and what they did. That can bring fresh insights. Some families turn to a respected elder, a clergyperson, or a medical professional who knows the situation, such as a palliative care specialist or longtime family doctor.

- **Get the help of a mediator**. Professional elder mediators are a terrific resource when big decisions (about where to live, how to spend money, or taking away the car keys) are tearing a family apart. Mediators cut stress and help families move forward by creating a safe and neutral space for all parties to be heard and for the interests of the person with dementia to be kept in view. They're also skilled at hammering out an action plan for a solution—so you don't just end the bickering but actually move forward. Mediators can be especially helpful where one party is crying foul louder than the others, or when suspicions about finances and motives have been raised.

Where can you find this family-saving expert? Ask your local Area Agency on Aging, a geriatric care manager, or lawyer to recommend mediators who specialize in eldercare or gerontology. They're typically family law attorneys.

Or check the Eldercare Locator, a service of the U.S. Administration on Aging. You'll spend a little money (rates average around $150/hour, depending where you live) but can actually save in the end when you face thorny money matters, not to mention priceless peace of mind and family harmony.

o o o

Strained Relationships

Some common scenarios:

Honor thy parent or thy partner first? Caring for a parent with dementia can take a lot of time—leaving one's spouse to feel resentful, even abandoned.

I am sandwich filling: While the average age of dementia caregivers is rising, many are women in their late 40s to early 50s—prime time to still have children in school along with aging parents (or a partner with early onset Alzheimer's). She feels constantly torn between the two generations. Men experience this, too. Children may complain of feeling neglected or begin to act out in ways that test limits.

Peter, Pammy, and Polly Pan: In a crisis, it's a typical dynamic for adult children to revert to their childhood roles and perceptions of one another. A successful lawyer born last remains the "baby" and sibs can't even take her legal advice seriously. Or the oldest is expected to make the hard decisions. Or the wild "black sheep" is left out of everything.

Family rifts: Caregiving situations can bring out ugly undercurrents with immediate or extended family. There may be disagreements about money, suspicions over motives, and disappointments over actions (or lack of actions).

Fair-weather friends: You get busy, they can't relate—and before you know it, there's a gulf between you and your friends. Or the idea of Alzheimer's scares them away.

What you should know about strained relationships:

Conflicts with the other people in your life are incredibly common. Alzheimer's doesn't just affect the person with the disease. Everyone in his or her circle is touched, as are, in turn, the relatives and friends in your circle.

Two-thirds of caregivers reported feeling isolated and alone in a 2017 Alzheimer's Association survey. At the same time, four-fifths of them wished they had more support and family help. Half don't feel they can talk at work or socially about what they're going through.

Half of caregivers also say that their duties take time away from friends and other family members, according to the National Alliance for Caregiving (NAC). And about a third of caregivers say that their emotions interfere "a lot" with their social lives, found a 2011 UCLA Center for Health Policy report. Fully 80 percent of caregivers report that caregiving strained their marriage or other key relationships, found a 2009 Caring.com survey.

And it all happens almost without you realizing it. "The risk of caregiving is that you gravitate toward newness—you have to pay attention to every new situation or crisis," says Carol D. O'Dell, author of *Mothering Mother*, who took care of her mom for 10 years. "And you ignore all the quieter people and situations in your life."

Net result: isolation, tension, resentment, a perceived lack of support, lost sources of support—and a lot more stress in an already overstressed life. Caregivers who sacrifice time with family and friends are more than twice as likely to feel stress as those who preserve time with others, according to NAC data.

What can help you:

- **Consciously decide that others matter**. This is a problem where sheer awareness helps. It's easy to get so focused on Alzheimer's that you take others for granted. In a crisis, that's inevitable. But you can't let crisis become chronic, because everyone needs you to some extent—and you need them. Keep a mental tally of the people who matter, and make a point of checking in. It never pays to take someone for granted for too long—including (especially) a beloved spouse.

- **Talk about your distraction**. Let others know that you know your presence has been scarce or conflicted. Try saying things like, "I can tell you're not happy now, and neither am I. I know things can't be exactly the same as they once were between us, right now, but let's work together to try harder."

- **Set up rituals that bring you together**. When your time and attention are at a premium, it can help to "institutionalize" together time. Make it part of your daily routine. Maybe you get up early to have breakfast with your teen before school or take an after-dinner walk with your spouse while your mom dozes.

- **Avoid making false assumptions**. When you're deep in dementia care, others' issues and interests can seem trivial by comparison. To you, perhaps they are. But they're not to the person having them. Make a concerted effort to ask about the challenges and concerns facing others in your life. Stay in the game—maybe not to your usual extent but enough to show you care. If you can't have a weekly lunch date, you can text or send birthday cards, for example.

- **Play fair**. Friendship is a two-way street. Try to make sure every conversation doesn't revolve around your dementia dramas and caregiving complaints.

- **Avoid forming unrealistic expectations**. It would be nice if everyone understood how difficult and consuming dementia care can be. But they don't. Even a long-loved spouse who lives under the same roof as you may not be completely on the same page. A teenager may adore Grandpa, but developmentally, it's normal for her to see herself as the center of her own universe, not her grandfather. Accept that these differences are not only okay but normal, and let them go. If you're constantly expecting people to pitch in or lend an ear in ways they're not, you'll be disappointed and nursing a hurt.

- **Outgrow old expectations**. Is someone locked into thinking a younger sibling is too immature to make decisions (even though she's 35)? Or that a son should manage money while a daughter manages doctor appointments? Gender stereotypes and childhood roles can get in the way of having good relationships now. Gently remind someone stuck in this kind of thinking that you're all grown-ups now.

- **Find solace in those who "know."** Support groups or online chat groups can be a kind of pressure valve for your primary relationships. When you can blow off steam to those who do know what you're going through, you're apt to be more emotionally available to, and more tolerant of, these other loved ones.

- **Sometimes, you just have to let 'em go**. It's not unusual for some friends or family to fall away due to the stress of caregiving. You might reunite later, or you might not. If a relationship can't stand up to being on the back burner temporarily, or if arguments are too corrosive, step back. Let the relationship die a natural death. Just be cautious not to do this with all your relationships simply because it feels easier. You need a support network now more than ever. Even when you're stressed, connection works both ways.

o o o

EMOTIONAL STRESSORS

When You Feel Guilty

Some common scenarios:

Guilt for what I'm not doing: I should be entertaining Grandma more...I need to cook healthier meals...I ought to get us both exercising....

Guilt for what I'm doing: I feel bad that I take him to the day center, but I need a break...I shouldn't rush through her shower like that...I ought to be able to handle this without whining. After all, I'm her daughter!

Guilt for not doing enough: After years of struggles, one caregiver agonized over whether it was time to place her diabetic and demented mom, who was obese and becoming incontinent, into a care facility. When her mom needed an amputation, the discharge planner and doctors agreed there was little question that this would be best. A good option was found that worked out well all around. But the caregiver couldn't help feeling that she'd let her mother down. "I feel like there's more I could have done...."

Guilt for being away: Long-distance caregivers feel their cash and phone support isn't enough. Those who use respite care are pricked with feelings of insufficiency when they can't do it 24/7.

Guilt for being happy or well: I'm in a good mood today. Oh wait, I shouldn't be, because my husband is sick. Why am I the healthy one and he's in such terrible shape?

What you should know about guilt:

As the examples illustrate, there's no end to opportunities for guilt in the realm of caregiving. You can't ignore this pesky emotion. You can't will it away. Guilt simply is.

Occasionally, guilt can be a productive emotion. Call it "good guilt"—the nagging voice in our heads that causes us to examine our behavior and decide whether a change is in order.

If you feel guilty because you were impatient with your loved one, for example, it's like a little poke reminding you to try harder or take a deep breath next time. Feeling guilty because you didn't go to the gym? Yes, that would have been good for you, and what would make that possible?

Unfortunately, most of what eats us alive is "bad guilt." Bad guilt has no constructive underbelly. Bad guilt makes you feel bad about a situation that you can't help (your parent has to move to rehab, for instance) or that is actually a positive for you (you've hired home care because you can't do it all yourself).

We beat ourselves up for reasons that are unrealistic and counterproductive. All that stewing and self-flagellation wastes precious mental energy.

(If you're a mother, you're probably a champion at guilt. Women who are actively being caregiving to both a parent and children at the same time are the overloaded filling of triple-decker guilt sandwiches.)

What can help you:

- **Beware the "red flag words"**: *Ought, should, could have, always, never.* Ban them from your vocabulary; they're warnings that you're setting the bar too high. When you hear yourself saying, "I should..." flick your forefinger against your wrist as a reminder. *Always* and *never* are toxic because they set us up for future guilt: "I'll never put you in a home." "I'll always be here." Avoid promising things you can't be 100 percent certain of—which is most things in life!

- **Don't discount yourself.** Ironically, selfless people (the dominant caregiver personality) tend to feel proportionately more guilt. Because they work so hard aspiring to an ideal of doing things for others, they tend to ignore the inconvenient reality that they have to look after themselves all the more. They may even forget that they, too, deserve extras and shortcuts and breaks. When they finally get around to a slow bath or a lunch with friends, it feels as alien as it does great. Trust your needs, your perceptions, your value in this situation.

- **Aim to be a B+ caregiver.** Straight A's are for grad students and crazoids, not mere mortals with houses to keep, relationships to tend, jobs to do, and sanity to uphold. No caregiver anticipates every fall or prevents every bedsore. Tempers boil. Germs sneak in. Bills slip through unpaid. In other words, life happens. No matter how much you love the person or feel you "owe" him or her, you'll all be happier if you lower your standards to the level of real life. By aiming for a B, you'll achieve good marks consistently, and occasionally surprise yourself with an A, rather than constantly feeling like you're missing the mark.

- **Remind yourself of your true goals here**. Ideally, you should be striving to help the person with dementia live a secure life free of worry or pain, while maintaining your own quality of life and health. Don't beat yourself up over the small stuff.

- **Steer clear of comparisons**. We feel guilt when we feel that we're falling short of some imagined ideal. Where do those ideas come from? Often, from inside our own head. We compare ourselves to someone else, without stopping to calculate what his or her stress levels or support situation is like, without allowing that every case is different. It doesn't matter if First Lady Nancy Reagan seemed like a saint about her husband's disease. Were you inside their house, seeing what went on? All that matters is you and yours, and how to make your hard situation as manageable as you can.

- **See enlisting help as a sign of strength, not weakness**. People who've been there know that dementia care is not a task for the isolated and solitary. The more you can delegate and share, the better life feels. Only those with too much pride and willful ignorance of reality think they can do it by themselves. Then when strong, savvy people get help, they don't look back and feel guilty about it.

- **Get the doctor's (or a therapist's) ten cents**. There's nothing like hearing a third party say, "No, you have nothing to feel guilty about in that situation." Often we don't believe the obvious unless we hear if from a trusted, neutral source.

Copy and post these promises to yourself:

1. I'll apologize when I lose my temper. But I'll also realize that caregiving is so full of temperature-rising situations that eternal calm is impossible.

2. I'll be there for my loved one, but also have to run my own life at the same time. Healthy caregiving is like staying balanced on a see-saw.

3. I'll let myself feel the full range of emotions—including grieving, crying, and feeling sad—instead of trying to keep a chipper smile on

my face all the time.

4. I'll accept or ignore criticism for what it's worth (or not worth) rather than letting it eat at me.

5. I'll quit blaming myself when bad things happen. Bad things happen.

6. I resolve to take care of me, not just my loved one. Because eventually I may be the one who needs care, and better it be later than sooner.

o o o

When You Feel Resentful

Some common scenarios:

Resenting others: "Why me?" You avoid Facebook because you're tired of reading about your friends' latest vacations and new cars. Relatives with big jobs go off to important offices every day. Everyone else seems to be living life to the fullest, while your days feel small and full of obligations.

Resenting fate: "Not the way it was supposed to be." "We were supposed to retire to the lake house." "I took care of the house and kids all those years, and now this was supposed to be my time." "I'm too young for this." "Other girls get to have their dads walk them down the aisle at their weddings; mine is in a nursing home with early onset Alzheimer's." "My wife spends all her time caring for her parents; what about me and our life?"

Resenting the person with dementia: "I love you and I hate you." "I'm just so tired of this." "Why didn't you take better care of yourself?" "Why didn't you tell me you were having trouble earlier?" "Why are you so difficult and ungrateful?" "Why do you blame me when I'm the one trying to help you?!"

What you should know about resentment:

Resentment is the "dirty little secret" emotion of caregiving. It's such a complex and taboo topic that few people readily cop to it. Yet it's an all-too-common feeling—and tends to ramp up the more hands-on the care you provide and the longer that caregiving goes on.

I can't tell you how many people come up to me when I speak on this topic and confide that they feel guilty about feeling this way.

Why shouldn't we resent a role none of us asked for and for which few of us have any real preparation? It's not only perfectly plausible, but natural, to love someone, care well for him or her, even continue to treasure moments together—and still resent the hijacked course your lives have taken because of this particularly insidious disease. Resentment can co-exist alongside other emotions.

For those who aren't close to the person who has dementia, or who don't have a long or happy history together, resentment can run especially high. I can testify to this firsthand.

Your life feels taken over. The situation feels endless. On top of that, you may be running without the reserves of goodwill that decades of happy memories can bring.

The dark side of resentment is that it can raise your blood pressure, shorten your temper, sap your energy, and lead you to drink, smoke, overeat, or relieve stress in other unhealthy ways. Not so good.

On the brighter side, having an awareness of your feelings—even the darkest ones—is the first step toward better health and can help improve your overall situation.

What can help you:

- **Start by acknowledging your resentment**. Give yourself permission to have this difficult emotion. It's okay. Resenting the fix you're in doesn't make you a bad person. It makes you a candid one.

- **Vent safely**. What's challenging about resentment is finding outlets that won't judge you or recoil in horror when you admit to it. A trusted friend to whom you can say anything is invaluable. Failing that, turn to support groups, a therapist, or online caregiver networks (where you can be anonymous if you prefer). Try scribbling your feelings in a journal. Then, if you want, rip them up or burn them afterward.

- **Try to avoid making comparisons**. This is really hard. Resentment tends to intensify when you compare one life to another—yours to your siblings' or friends', your past to your present, your long-dreamed future to your revised reality. When you catch yourself going there, pull back. Say it out loud: "I don't want to go there!"

- **Let yourself be galvanized, rather than paralyzed, by resentment**. Consider these prickly feelings as a personal message system. Use them as a warning that you should find more resources for help, enlist others in ways large and small, defend your health, and take other steps that will improve your day-to-day existence.

- **Identify the small things that bring you pleasure and seek them out**. Maybe you're more homebound than you'd like, but you treasure your garden. Maybe your spouse is suffering but your grandchildren bring joy. Make room for whatever treats you can muster, from an evening glass of wine or movie-channel subscription to a regular pedicure or video calls with an old friend.

- **Revisit the big picture every now and then**. A given hour, day, or week might be especially awful. Step back and look at the full arc of your life—past and future. It won't change what you're going through but can grant you a perspective that makes it more bearable.

o o o

When You Lose Your Temper or Patience

Some common scenarios:

Taking it out on your loved one: It used to startle me to hear my mother snap at my dad. When the phone rang, he might pick up one of the three TV remotes and say "Hello!" into it. (He had dementia, but those long black devices all looked similar!) "Not that one, the other one!" Mom would hiss at him—as if it hadn't happened a hundred times before.

Taking it out on a third party: Out of the blue, you yell at your child, just because she left her shoes on the floor. Or you call the girl at the drive-thru window a name because she forgot to put napkins in your bag. Told on the phone that you can't get your preferred appointment time, you erupt into full Mount MisplacedAngerSuvius.

What you should know about anger and impatience:

Everybody "loses it" sometimes. It may not be a particularly attractive human quality, but it's a natural act. In the setting of Alzheimer's caregiving, it might even be an inevitable one.

Anger often seems like it's being tripped by what's happening at the moment: a mistake, a balky loved one, a criticism, a mishap. But typically the incident is just the proverbial straw that breaks your back. There are usually underlying factors simmering beneath the surface. These can include chronic stress, lack of sleep, frustration over a lack of control, grief, or disappointments that have little direct connection to the meltdown.

"Stress rolls downhill" is how Oprah's favorite life coach, Martha Beck, refers to this displaced aggression. We tend to dump our anger on someone else, usually someone we know won't fight back.

Blowing up lets you release a little steam, momentarily. It's not the best way to let off steam, but it works—which is why we keep doing it.

Beware, though: Chronic anger and hostility are linked to high blood pressure, heart attack and heart disease, digestive tract disorders, and headaches. Anger that builds and doesn't get expressed can lead to depression or anxiety. Anger that explodes outwardly can jeopardize relationships and even cause harm. That's why finding good ways to manage caregiving impatience and anger helps both you and the person in your care.

What can help you:

When you slip:

- **For the occasional blooper, forgive yourself and forget**. Seriously.

- **Apologize to the injured party with a little self-blame**: "I'm so sorry. I don't know where that came from—well, I do; I've just been under a lot of stress. It's my fault, not yours." Or, "Sorry! That was the stress talking! It's about me, not you!"

- **Vow to try harder next time**. Patience really is a virtue, which is what makes it a worthy goal—even if not always an attainable one.

- **If you find yourself losing your patience constantly, consider it a wake-up call that you probably need more help**. Whether the stress is coming from loss of sleep, worry, frazzled nerves, or another source, you need relief. Look into adult day programs or hiring an elder companion. See if a relative will spell you for some set number of hours a day or week.

To avoid future slips:

- **If your anger is usually targeted at the person with dementia, remind yourself that he or she can't change**. You have to. Try to see the situation (confusing the phone and TV remote, endless repetition, moving slowly) from his or her perspective.

- **Try taking a few deep breaths at the moment you feel your fury rising**. You'd be surprised how quickly anger switches from one kind of biological response to another. (Some people get to a similar place via prayer.) More tactics when you feel the heat rising: Tackle a repetitive household chore that requires energy, like scouring pans, chopping vegetables, or mowing grass. Lift hand weights for a few reps.

Tip: **"When I lose it or feel myself about to, I chant to myself: 'It's okay, let it go.'"** —L.G.

- **Physically remove yourself from the situation for a moment**. Some caregivers have been known to excuse themselves to do a "silent scream" in the bathroom or a louder one in a car parked in the garage. Better yet: Practice preventative removal. Give yourself little breaks every couple of hours to have a cup of tea, look at the paper, sit outside and gaze at the sky.

- **Ask yourself if there's a constructive solution to situations that make you angry repeatedly**: Is compromise possible? Would being more assertive (which is different from anger) help you have a better sense of control?

- **Don't try to fit three errands in a two-errand time slot**. The math is against you. And make that one errand if the person with dementia is with you.

- **Vent better**. If you notice a pattern forming (or, ahem, if someone else points it out to you), look for some healthier outlets for your pent-up feelings. Maybe more exercise, or a different kind, would help. Could you confide in an online chat group? Write in a journal? Even if you burn it up or hit delete right after, research shows that getting the words out eases your burden.

o o o

When You Grieve (Even Though Your Loved One Is Alive)

Some common scenarios:

Mourning what once was: Reminders of the way your loved one used to be, before dementia, can be painful when you look at old photographs or bump into the person's former colleagues who ask he or she is doing.

Mourning what is now: Your loved one is alive, and yet every day brings new sad realities. Widowed friends tell you that "at least" your partner is still alive. Or is he? Alzheimer's isn't called "the longest goodbye" for nothing.

Mourning the future that will, and won't, be: A retirement bungalow in the country that won't happen. A long-saved-for cruise that won't be shared. A father who won't give a toast at his daughter's wedding. A grandchild who won't know her grandparent.

What you should know about grief:

The unique grief of those whose family member has dementia is every bit as real and intense as the type of mourning that takes place after a death. It consists of two different psychological states experienced at once, experts say:

1. *Anticipatory grief:* coping with very real feelings of loss for someone who is alive

2. *Ambiguous loss:* interacting with someone who's not fully present socially or mentally

Alzheimer's involves a series of losses: the loss of the ability to work, to drive, to cook, to read and write, to manage basic self-care, to engage fully with the world. Although we're encouraged by insightful experts to focus on what is, rather than what isn't, it's impossible to completely overlook this torrent of losses. We grieve each of them.

University of Indianapolis researchers asked more than 400 caregivers the open-ended question, "What would you say is the biggest barrier you have faced as a caregiver?" More than eight in ten referred to the loss of the person they used to know.

What can help you:

- **Please know that your feelings are normal**. It can help simply to know that anticipatory grief exists. Don't fall into the trap of thinking that because a loved one is still alive, you aren't entitled to dark emotions. Nor does it make any sense that you should be expected to hold them in.

- **Let go of associated guilt**. People often feel guilty for experiencing the difficult feelings that go along with anticipatory grief and ambiguous loss. But they're very real and logical emotions. Why wouldn't a reasonable person be sad and mournful about the great changes at hand? True, someone with dementia is still "here," but we all know it's possible to be both here and not here, in Alzheimer's World.

- **Understand that it's real grief**. A 2001 study in the journal *The Gerontologist* described anticipatory grief as equivalent in intensity and breadth to the response to death. The odd silver lining: Anticipatory grief prepares us for the eventual end. It's a long, slow, painful warm-up, but it is a warm-up. (Not that you'll be fully inoculated against intense sadness and mourning later.)

- **Stay realistic about how hard dementia care is**. Many caregivers wax poetic about those unexpected "I love you" moments or sudden bursts of clarity and gratitude. You're likely to hear people talk this way at support groups, online, or in books. Such moments are fulfilling and should be embraced, by all means. But the rest of the time—well, there's the rest of the time. Don't beat yourself up if you struggle with some aspects of caregiving.

- **Be nice to yourself**. Grief (anticipatory or otherwise) puts you at risk for depression. Depression puts you at risk for dementia. How to get off this vicious cycle? Start small. Enlist a regular volunteer or paid aide to take over while you do something positive for your own health, such as working out. Make self-care a priority in your day. Caring and self-caring are intimately related.

- **Rely on a support network for an emotional outlet**. You may feel the need to put on a "brave face" in front of the sick person all the time, when expressing your conflicting feelings is what would serve you better. A support network lets you do that. Spousal caregivers can have a tougher time getting out and connecting with friends and relatives, especially if you have health issues yourself. Yet spouses are at greater risk for depression. Venting on paper—writing about your feelings—can help during those moments when you can't see someone face to face. Long-term studies have found that Alzheimer's caregivers who receive counseling and support, formal or informal, have better health and a lower incidence of depression.

- **Consider a legacy project**. Many families are buoyed, or at least distracted, from the pain of loss by actively celebrating the life of the person with Alzheimer's. Sample projects include recording an audiovisual life story (in the mild to moderate stages), pulling together a scrapbook or photo album, writing a biography, or organizing and documenting a collection or other endeavor representative of the person's life. It doesn't have to be a life record. A legacy project can also be the creation of something the person leaves behind—a joke book for grandchildren, lap robes knit for charity, donating a special collection to the right place, marching in an Alzheimer's walk as a family team.

  Transforming feelings of pain into pride and meaning, a legacy project is also a terrific distraction that helps you feel productive.

- **Explore hospice**. Eventually, the person in your care will reach end-stage dementia (or succumb to another illness first). Finding out about hospice programs near you, and what they entail, isn't a secret death wish, as some people mistakenly believe. You can't control the timing of the end. But it does come, and you deserve the skilled guidance that experts in this passage can offer you, even if it's still months or years in the unknowable future. See: Chapter 5, "End-of-Life Care."

o o o

PRACTICAL STRESSORS

Lack of Privacy

Some common scenarios:

Not the Waltons: Unlike TV's Appalachia-poor Walton family—night after night, everyone sits in the cramped family room arguing over what to watch on TV. At dinner, the conversation is tense and strained as Grandpa struggles to get the food in his mouth and the kids can't wait to snarf and split.

Not the Golden Girls: Your parent moved in—and now expects to do everything with you. Or your spouse has become overly clingy, following you everywhere.

Not the stuff of home movies, either: Your mom thinks nothing of walking into your bedroom, even when the door is shut. Dad riffles through the papers on your desk while you're at work, and you can't find anything. When you go to the bathroom, your grandmother knocks—every time—asking, "Are you in there? Is anybody in there?"

What you should know about privacy:

Everyone in a caregiving family needs the freedom to exist in his or her own space. Having physical privacy means having boundaries that let everyone in the household escape 24/7 interactions. This is especially challenging in small living spaces.

It's easy for even loving families to feel way too close for comfort. The person with dementia may need help with basic needs, from meal planning to toileting. Disinhibition (loss of social appropriateness) may lead him or her to barge into bedrooms and bathrooms, or say and do embarrassing things in front of guests. Or you may be shadowed closely wherever you go.

It's not just your sanity at stake. You also need the privacy to be able to continue with some version of long-established family time and traditions, important both now and far into the future. With a live-in parent or grandparent, you ideally weave them into the existing family life, while balancing the need for kids and spouse to have their own routines and share of your attention.

What can help you:

- **Create to-each-his-own spaces**. Ideally a live-in elder has his or her own living quarters, not just for sleeping but also for living. See if their bedroom might be able to hold a TV and comfortable chair, a desk, even (in a perfect world) a private bathroom and a small refrigerator or kitchenette. Sometimes minor home improvements can deliver what you need. My brother turned a hall closet next to a bedroom into an en-suite bathroom.

- **Explore whether a parent's assets can be used to fund a modest addition to your home**. Some families discover that this is a cheaper alternative to out-of-home care. It can also increase the value of the home.

- **Preserve non-elder time**. Remain conscious of maintaining one-on-one time with other family members. There's no rule that says your live-in parent must always come first with you, go out to dinner with you, or join you on family vacations. Use respite care or other relatives to supplement care.

- **Get physically away**. Everyone in the house needs opportunities to get away, especially a hands-on caregiver. Don't put vacations, school or sports events, or other routine family activities on indefinite hold.

- **Don't be afraid to use locks**. When someone with dementia begins to invade your private space, logic and kind requests will do little good. Install simple deadbolts in your bedroom and master bath. (You'll still get interrupted but without the intrusion.)

  Locks in bathrooms are trickier because you don't want the person to accidentally lock himself in and be unable to get out. Experts often recommend removing bathroom locks for this reason. One option: locks that can be opened from either side. These may be tricky enough to keep the person out but still allow you to go in, if needed. Plastic doorknob covers that are hard to grip can also deter someone from entering rooms.

- **Remember that kids need space, too**. Avoid making a child share a room with an elder if at all possible. While family togetherness is nice, don't force caregiving responsibilities. It doesn't help anyone if a child nurses resentment.

- **If boundary-intruding becomes overwhelming**: Mention these behaviors to the doctor, especially if they take a sudden change for the more insistent. Medication interactions or alcohol use can worsen behaviors, or there may be another underlying cause. Eventually, for your own health and your loved one's safety, you may not be able to live under one roof.

o o o

Lack of "Me" Time

Some common scenarios:

Feeling like a hermit: You used to have a social life. You went to book club, met people for dinner or the odd dishy lunch. You got your hair done, instead of pulling it back into an ever-longer ponytail. Now, you can't even remember when you last visited the mall, meandering at your own pace.

Feeling unfit: You hear about the importance of exercise and self-care over and over, but who has time to get to the gym? Heck, who has time—since you can't leave your loved one home alone—to walk around the block? And if you bring her with you, it means getting all the aerobic output of a snail.

Feeling like a stranger to yourself: There's no time for reading a Twitter feed, much less the latest novel. Some days, you feel you can barely hear yourself think. Your own thoughts don't seem to matter, anyway, crowded out as they are by worries, doctor appointments, medication reminders, toileting reminders, drink-more-water-Dad reminders.

What you should know about taking time for yourself:

Though everyone values the idea of "me" time, many caregivers are convinced they can't find any. It's not easy, but it's always possible. Dream big. Start small.

You'll be better able to weather stress. Have more energy. Think more clearly. Feel less overwhelmed. Better avert depression. Be healthier and able to provide better care, longer.

What can help you:

- **Yes, start small:** Aim for just 10 or 15 minutes daily if you feel it's hopeless. Literally write what you'll do on your planner or daily to-do list. Commit to carving this same time out every day. (Don't plan to randomly grab 15 minutes whenever you can.) Life coaches say it can take up to three weeks for a new habit to take hold. Devoting specific times to yourself helps you make "me" time a priority. What can you do in just 10 or 15 minutes that will make a difference? Pump free weights (start with two- or three-pound dumbbells). Write a note or text a friend you miss. Make a playlist of your favorite high-energy or sing-along tunes and crank them up. Music with a strong beat is known to boost energy; orchestral and acoustic music can improve thinking.

- **Schedule time for yourself early in your day**. Don't make personal time an afterthought or reward after you finish the day's business. Mark out "you" time early in the day, so the day doesn't run away from you. Plus, you'll be better able to face the day if you're more energized.

- **Make the break feel like an indulgence**. No laundry. No paying the bills. Think of something you enjoyed when you had more time, before your life got crazy. Maybe it's savoring flavored tea in a china cup while reading a brand-new book you've downloaded. Maybe it's setting up a craft table to pursue a project you've abandoned.

- **Now go broader**: After a week or so of adding a daily break, block out a larger span of time at least weekly to do something self-indulgent away from home. Get a massage or a manicure, take a walk in a nearby park, attend a book group.

Tip: **"I make time for prayer every morning. It's something I've always done, but now I treasure the time more than ever—to ask for strength and then feel calm and ready for anything after. I think meditation or yoga or whatever your source of spiritual strength is would do the same if you do it early and every day." —E.F.**

- **Just say, "No."** If you're tempted to yield to a request, get in the habit of replying, "I'm not sure; let me get back to you." Even if you're pretty sure you're able to do it, don't answer immediately. Give yourself a cushion of time to reflect privately on whether the request will enhance your life or detract from it. Saying "no" is like working a muscle. The more you express regrets or bow out, the easier it becomes the next time.

If you find it hard to refuse others (and this is true for many people with caregiver hearts), rehearse a few lines to fall back on: "I'd love to help, but I just have too much going on right now." Or, "I wish I could, but it will have to be another time." Humor helps: "If I take on even one more thing, my husband will divorce me and my hair will catch on fire."

Be especially protective if indulging a favor or taking on a new task would nip into your personal time. You'll never find enough time for yourself if you don't cordon it off.

- **Create a "you" cave**. It could be a whole spare bedroom or a desk and comfy chair in a corner. Decorate your "me zone" with meaningful mementos, a comfy quilt, your favorite photos.

  Having your own personal retreat ensures you'll be more likely to head there to do something just for yourself—watch a DVD, Skype with an old high school pal, run through some yoga moves, take a power nap. Ask others in the house to respect your privacy when you're in your personal space. (It doesn't always work, but it never hurts to ask!)

- **Try a portable "you" zone**. When you can't get to your special space, or can't create one, and you're feeling overwhelmed, remember that you can clear a "me zone" in your head. Close your eyes and take a few calming deep breaths. Some people find it helpful to retreat to the bathroom to get this kind of privacy. Or do a "mind sweep": Jot down all the things troubling you (conflicts, to-do items). The simple act of making a list releases some of the tension and helps you prioritize.

- **Share your load**. Spend less time on things that don't absolutely require your personal involvement by delegating, rotating, or outsourcing. For most families, even when one person is the primary caregiver, giving care is a family-wide experience. Is there anyone in your household who can make dinner one night a week? Run a vacuum? Cut the lawn? Enlist kids as well as adults. Perhaps one person could clean up as you cook, reducing the need for a big clean after. Post a chore schedule, with everybody taking a shift. Look into sharing the marketing or a carpool with a neighbor. Consider a "parent-sitting" exchange with a friend who also has a live-in elderly parent who can't stay alone.

- **Don't discount the person with dementia as a helper**. Don't do things for older relatives that they can still do for themselves. Too often, families err on the side of "helping" to excess. Until late-stage Alzheimer's, activities such as cleaning or folding laundry can provide the person with a healthful sense of usefulness and contribution.

It's fine to work side-by-side if the person wouldn't be safe working alone. But resist the urge to help, hover, or take over because the job isn't meeting your standards. Figure out which things you can let go.

- **Look for shortcuts and other streamlining efficiencies**. For one whole day, analyze the way you do all your routine tasks with an eye toward saving time. For example, paying bills online is faster than writing checks, stuffing envelopes, scrambling for stamps, and mailing them. It's a tiny time difference, but the saved minutes add up.

  Could you make lunches every other day, preparing two at a time? Or make a casserole or pot of soup you can heat up for several days running? Plan errands for times of day when crowds are thinner (avoiding lunchtime and rush hour, for example). Scheduling morning medical appointments, or the first appointment after lunch, means less waiting-room time, because the doctor is less likely to have gotten backed up.

- **Tackle the dregs first**. Try to get your least favorite or hardest tasks out of the way early in the day, when you have more energy. That way you'll chip through more pleasant jobs during the rest of the day with a sense of accomplishment, rather than energy-draining dread.

  Or double up: Pair a task you don't like with one you do. Iron or run on the treadmill while you catch up on a pre-recorded or streamed favorite TV show or reach out to a friend by cell phone to chat (and vent as needed!). If you're paying bills online, open up a second window to chat with fellow caregivers in an online forum. Download new books or magazines onto your phone or tablet, so you can skip taking the time to go to the library or bookstore. Bonus: You'll always have escapist reading material at your fingertips in doctors' waiting rooms, on the bus, in between errands.

- **Take mini-breaks**. We all need more escapes than we can get in a day or week. Try an occasional quick fix throughout your day. Paced deep breathing is known to lower heart rate and blood pressure. Or treat yourself to a square of dark chocolate. Yes, it can actually lower stress hormones, according to a Swiss (where else?) study, which gave people a two-inch square every day for two weeks. Half was eaten at mid-morning and half at mid-afternoon. (Don't beat yourself up if you can't make it last that long.)

A neat de-stressing trick: Relive a "memory snapshot." The next time you're having a wonderful experience—a birthday party, a quiet walk by yourself in a beautiful place, a simple interaction with your loved one—imprint the memory on your mind by focusing intently on everything you can about the moment, using all of your senses. What do you see up close and all around you? Take in the colors, the textures, the details. What does it smell like? What does a piece of chocolate cake taste like? Spending just 30 seconds consciously taking in as much as you can about a moment helps imprint it on your brain, making the full experience easier to recall later. Then, when you're stressed, close your eyes and conjure up the memory you "photographed." It's a quickie escape that can recapture the positive feelings you had in that moment—and bring them into your present.

- **Unplug**. As much as electronic gadgets help us multitask, they can also become time-suckers that lead us to squander downtime moments we didn't realize we hand. That's how we wind up zoning in front of the TV all evening (watching something we don't even like) or flipping through catalogs and social media threads for hours and yet never feeling like we have time to ourselves.

  Try starting with 15 "silent" minutes a day. If it plugs in, unplug it or turn it off. You don't necessarily have to spend that time on yourself to feel like you've gained something. The quality of your interactions with others will seem deeper when you focus more on one another. Your psyche comes away refreshed without the chronic distraction of competing interests.

- **Buy time**. Don't underestimate the value of outsourcing. Yes, it means spending money. But your time carries a price tag, too—and your health and peace of mind are priceless. Weigh the costs of a biweekly cleaning service against the time you spend on such tasks now. Look into a grocery delivery service or take-out meals, which many supermarkets now offer. Pay a neighborhood kid to handle yard work and to clean gutters. Hire a teenager to relieve you every afternoon at five for an hour, so you can take an exercise class. (Ask a local Scout troop or high school for reliable candidates.) Look for freelance handyman or errand services in your area, like TaskRabbit. A free option: local church youth groups or schools, which often require students to earn service hours by helping those in need.

Professional caregivers, from nurse aides to elder companions, can help in the home. Adult day programs, for those able to attend them, are another source of "found hours" for you and a win-win, since most people are energized by attending them.

- **Don't be shy about asking for the gift of time**. If your budget is stretched, consider asking relatives who have offered to help if they'll pay for specific kinds of relief. Many of us hate to "talk money," but long-distance caregivers who can't give their time often welcome such an opportunity to feel like they're making a difference. And when someone asks what you want for your birthday or a holiday, or what the person with dementia needs, ask for the gift of time (or the money to buy it).

The trick is to apply the time you buy toward yourself, not anything or anyone else. If an aide or a sibling spends time with your loved one on Saturday mornings, go out to do something personally meaningful during that block of time. Don't just run errands. By having short breaks from each other, you and the person you're caring for will both be more apt to come together again stimulated by the change and—critical for you—renewed.

o o o

Your Own Sleep Problems (Insomnia, Sleep Deprivation)

Some common scenarios:

Kept awake by worry: Whether the topic is money, care logistics, work, or any of 1,000 other concerns on your plate, ruminating in the dark is a sure path to insomnia.

Disrupted by Alzheimer's: If the person keeps getting up to use the bathroom or pace the halls, chances are your sleep cycle will be disrupted, too. When day and night are completely mixed up due to dementia, the whole household can suffer.

Burning the candle at both ends: There are only so many hours to do soooooo many things. Many caregivers rise extra early and stay up extra late. The house is quiet, but this "found time" is stolen from sleep.

Body gone haywire: Caregivers tend to be mid-lifers or older, ages when our own bodies experience problems that can disrupt sleep, separate from dementia care. On this list: menopause, bladder problems, prostate problems, thyroid disorders, restless leg syndrome, sleep apnea, and medication interactions, to name a few.

What you should know about sleep problems:

Sleep scientists now know that getting enough good-quality sleep is a linchpin to overall health and stress levels. Sleep is protective against disorders ranging from obesity to heart disease—and dementia! Sleep boosts mood. Sleep gives energy. Sleep helps us organize our memories and protects brain function. Far from being useless downtime into which you should cram laundry, paperwork, and computer surfing, night hours should be your best friend in your quest to provide good quality care for as long as possible. In short, you can't get along very well, or go very far, without sleep.

The irony is that caregivers often ignore their own disturbed or insufficient sleep because it just doesn't seem as critical as all the other fires that need putting out in a day. Or it may feel like an insurmountable problem.

What can help you:

In general:

- **Know that if dementia-disrupted sleep is the root cause, you must address it**. Families too often excuse or ignore sleep problems in the person they look after. There are two main reasons, says geriatric psychiatrist Ken Robbins. First, they mistakenly assume that poor sleep is just part of aging, or part of dementia, and think nothing can be done about it. Second, they fear that making a big issue about it and seeking medical help is just a selfish act—as if the sleep problem were only theirs, and not a shared one. Solving sleep problems helps everyone.

- **Be honest about other symptoms**. Along with feeling tired and draggy, do you notice other physical changes that you've been ignoring? A racing pulse? Feeling out of breath on stairs? A leaky bladder when you laugh or sneeze? Sleep may be related to another health issue you should have checked out now by your doctor. Don't just complain about your sleep. Take inventory of anything else bothering you, and report it.

Waking up tired even after you think you've slept is a key warning sign of sleep apnea, a common (and fortunately treatable) condition that causes people to miss breaths while they sleep.

Before going to bed:

- **Get the basics down**. You may not be able to control when you're awakened, but at least you can structure an environment that's pro-sleep. These are the same tips as for someone with dementia who awakens: The bedroom should be cool, quiet, and dark. Take out the TV. Don't play the radio or use devices there (the blue light will keep you up). Change into sleep clothes; even if you prefer sweats or lounge PJ's, make them items you wear only for bed, not for daytime, too.

- **Try over-the-counter sleep aids for a few nights**. They can help you restore your sleep cycle and get needed rest. If you feel you need to use them more than a few nights a week for more than a few weeks, that's a sign you should have yourself checked out. Your doctor may also be able to prescribe a stronger sleep medicine to reset your sleep cycle. Some caregivers swear by melatonin, a hormone sold at drugstores.

- **Pick the right nightcap**. Alcohol? No—it will help you nod off but then awaken you later as it moves through your system. Warm milk—yes. The amino acid it contains really does help to calm you. Avoid caffeine crutches (coffee, tea, cocoa) after early afternoon.

- **Eat for sleep**. Oatmeal before bed can elevate your blood sugar in a way that triggers sleep-inducing brain chemicals and keeps blood sugar steady, so you can sleep. Oats also contain vitamin B6 and melatonin, which promote relaxation. Bananas are another source of melatonin, as well as serotonin. Go for the sleep-lulling trifecta: oatmeal made with milk and topped with banana.

- **Think calming down, not revving up**. If you're having sleep trouble, avoid exercising at night. Instead try gentle stretching, meditation, yoga, or relaxation moves. A good example of the latter: Systematically clench and release each major muscle group, starting at your forehead and moving down to your toes. Avoid scheduling family conference calls or updates to relatives late in the day before bed if these conversations risk riling you up.

When you wake up at night:

- **Don't blend day and night yourself**. When you do get up at night, keep the room dark. Leave the room to read or sit up awake until you feel sleepy.

- **Try this trick that helps ruminators who can't stop their thoughts from racing**: Keep a notebook on your bedside table. Write down what you're thinking about. Committing the worrisome thoughts—or a possible to-do list—to paper can help you jettison it from your brain for a while, so you can rest.

- **Repeat the evening relaxers**. Have a glass of warm milk. Do progressive relaxation exercises. Avoid the TV, tablet, and phone.

More help:

- **Practice the power nap**. The good news about naps is that they're linked to lower blood pressure, less heart disease, healthy weight, more energy, and improved mood— the same benefits as nighttime sleep. An oft-quoted study in the journal *Sleep* pinpointed the ideal nap length at 10 minutes. Sleep more than 30 minutes and you start to cycle into sleep stages that mean you'll wake up feeling groggy, not refreshed.

One trick: The caffeine nap. Have a cup of coffee about 20 minutes before a short nap. It takes about half an hour for caffeine to kick in. So shortly after you wake up, the java will jolt, leaving you doubly energized.

- **Consider p.m. respite care**. If you absolutely need to sleep at night, try hiring a night nurse or aide to be on duty at least a few nights a week. Even if the person with dementia doesn't always get up at night, just knowing that someone else is in charge for a few hours can provide the peace of mind you need to fall into deep and restorative slumber.

o o o

"The time of life we call dying is an extremely difficult part of the life cycle, but a normal part. The nature of it isn't medical, it's experiential."

—Ira Byock, MD, palliative-care medicine advocate

5: END-OF-LIFE CARE

Help for the final stage of dementia caregiving

You're welcome to—really, I urge you to—read this chapter at any point in your caregiving journey. Given that dementia is a condition that steadily erodes the brain, body, and personality, it would be unusual not to wonder long in advance about what to expect toward the end and what you can do. Others prefer to wait until they're there, and that's normal, too.

Despite good days and gratifying moments (and as hard as it is to come to terms with this), someone with significant dementia has been slowly dying before your eyes for some time. Looking ahead and seeking answers is both natural and healthy. Even "long goodbyes" come to a final farewell.

Some consider it unseemly or even "jinx-y" to think preemptively about death. To the contrary, it's almost always more helpful for everyone involved. For you and your family, knowing what's normal now can help you brace emotionally, put practical plans in place, make medical decisions with more confidence, and bring comfort right to the end.

For the person with dementia, your insights can mean better and more compassionate care and greater odds of the "good death" that most people desire, even if they can't put it into words.

It's a fraught time. Throughout Alzheimer's care, you already experience a kind of grieving, and this grief—along with surreal confusion, worry, even guilt-laced relief—can intensify as the end draws closer. One silver lining to the kind of mourning happening now: Psychologist Barry Jacobs, author of *The Emotional Survival Guide for Caregivers*, describes it as paving the way for more productive grieving later, featuring less guilt and concern over whether you did right by your relative.

As is true of so much that's characteristic of dealing with Alzheimer's and other dementias, all of these intense feelings are okay. We're only human.

This section considers the practical and emotional issues you may encounter toward the end of the life of someone with dementia. It's a poignant time that demands frank advice.

o o o

HOW WILL I KNOW?

Life Expectancy

People especially search for answers to this question at the outset of diagnosis and again late into the disease: How long can someone with Alzheimer's or another dementia be expected to live?

Unfortunately, what's known is only somewhat useful to any specific case. The Alzheimer's Association puts average life expectancy at 4 to 8 years after diagnosis. The Mayo Clinic cites 8 to 10 years. And most everyone notes that it can be as long as 20 years. For vascular dementia and dementia with Lewy bodies, average life expectancy tends to be slightly less.

Research shows that three variables seem to lead to shorter lifespans with dementia:

1. *Age when the first symptoms appeared.* Higher age means shorter duration. In one analysis, someone diagnosed at 65 lives an average of 9 years, vs. 3 years at age 90.

2. *Gender.* Women tend to live slightly longer.

3. *The level of impairment at diagnosis.* The worse the symptoms are at the start, the quicker the finish.

Not that averages make your particular crystal ball any less cloudy.

More concretely, it's possible to recognize when an individual is moving into the final stage of dementia (or another illness).

Recognizing End-stage Dementia

End-stage (terminal) dementia is the final weeks to months of life for someone who has already reached the severe/advanced stage. Basically, the physical degeneration caused by Alzheimer's disease or another dementia gets bad enough that the person almost inevitably starts to experience life-threatening problems like repeated pneumonias or other infections.

End-stage dementia typically lasts under a year in total, rarely more than two years.

By the time it begins, the person has already been living in a state where they:

- Require total help with bathing, dressing, and grooming

- Have bladder and possibly bowel incontinence
- Are no longer able to self-feed (although will still open the mouth and eat if cued by spoon-feeding)
- Are likely bedbound and unable to walk
- Sleep a lot
- Show little meaningful communication (talk less, are more difficult to understand) and may not recognize family

Someone can live for years in this state, where "the mind seems gone but the body remains able enough to keep living, as long as food and a safe, supportive environment are provided," says geriatrician and geriatrics health educator Leslie Kernisan, MD, of BetterHealthWhileAging.net.

Eventually, Alzheimer's kills by weakening the brain and the body, including the immune system and motor function. The person becomes more vulnerable to things like:

- Pneumonia, the leading cause of dementia deaths (as many as half of all people with advanced dementia develop pneumonia in the last two weeks of life)
- Other infections, such as kidney infections or septicemia (infections in the bloodstream)
- Continuing and severe pressure ulcers (bed sores), especially those that persist despite adequate wound care and proper positioning
- Eating problems, such as being unable to swallow, pocketing food in the cheek, refusal to eat or drink
- Significant weight loss (because the person can't or won't eat, or the body can no longer absorb nutrients): about 5 percent or more within one month, or unexpected weight loss over three or more months
- Blood clots, from being bedridden

When these events begin to happen, the likelihood that the person will die within months, not years, goes way up. Infections (including pneumonia), fevers, and eating problems are the most certain signs that a person who has very advanced dementia will die within 12 to

18 months, a 2009 *New England Journal of Medicine* investigation found.

Other Causes of Death in Someone With Dementia

The older the person, the more likely other chronic diseases are also at work. Many people with dementia succumb first to something other than dementia, such as heart disease or cancer. Or someone whose Alzheimer's is transitioning from moderate to severe might go into a rapid downward spiral after a hospitalization for a hip fracture or another serious health shock. For example, a fall leads to surgery, immobility, a further decline in cognitive function, and pneumonia.

Sometimes the final downturn comes in one dramatic change. More often there's a rollercoaster of declines and rallies that might be launched by a catastrophic event. Also common: "the dwindles," when a person slowly weakens away.

When any of these scenarios begin before advanced dementia, the person may be more lucid and mobile than the symptoms described in the previous section, almost to the end.

My dad, for example, had vascular dementia for years. While still in its moderate stage, a minor stroke landed him in the hospital, then four months in rehabilitation in a long-term care facility's dementia wing, where he died at age 87. But the official cause of death was kidney cancer.

In my father-in-law's case, his fairly robust health wobbled gradually over the last two years of his life before a sudden final nosedive. Was it simply the advancing dementia? The congestive heart failure he'd had for more than a decade? Ongoing effects of an earlier stroke that an MRI had revealed? Something else? All of the above? Doctors found it hard to say. He was 95.

One way that doctors and nurses know a person is turning a corner to the end is when he or she shows signs of cachexia, the metabolic syndrome of "wasting away": extreme weight loss, muscle loss, fatigue, and loss of strength. Cachexia features in almost every end-stage major illness—not only in dementia but also cancer, heart failure, kidney disease, Crohn's disease, rheumatoid arthritis, and others.

Here's a good place to emphasize that hospice care can make an enormous difference during this final stage. Later sections in this chapter will cover what you should know about hospice as well as other guidance on navigating end-of-life care, including the specific signs of when death is very close.

o o o

PLANNING AHEAD

A major challenge for you now is how to manage shifting care needs in ways that best preserve comfort and dignity, provide relief from pain, and minimize emotional distress—for someone who's almost never able to weigh in. While much of caring for someone with advanced dementia feels reactive (something happens, we scramble to respond), there are some important things you can think about ahead of time as well as in that moment that will help shape your actions.

A key thing to realize is this: the usual "default" for the medical system, including among many of those who staff memory care units and nursing homes, is to do everything necessary to treat illness and prevent death.

That's why studies show that many people with advanced dementia—far too many, it can reasonably be argued—experience hospitalizations and sometimes even surgeries or other invasive procedures in the last months of their life. It's not necessarily bad or wrong when this happens, but it's not always good, either. In many places, the pendulum is swinging away from thinking that "do everything" medically is inevitably in every patient's best interests.

The best scenario is when families understand all of their options ahead of time and can work with doctors to proactively choose a plan of care that's a good fit with their loved one's preferences and health situation.

You can get ahead on that curve by considering these main questions:

Consider: What Would the Person Want?

In an ideal world, medical preferences for end-of-life care are spelled out in written documents—such as a living will—made when your loved one still had the legal capacity to make decisions.

There may also be medical directives known in different states as POLST (provider orders for life-sustaining treatment), MOLST (medical orders for life-sustaining treatment), POST (physician's orders on scope of treatment), and MOST (medical orders on scope of treatment). Usually on a single sheet of bright paper, these documents are increasingly being used. They summarize patient-provider conversations about treatment preferences and are designed to travel with a patient from setting to setting (such as home to hospital or nursing home) and to be followed by all medical staff.

POLST-type orders should be in the medical record. Be sure all advance directive documents are easily accessible. Get them out of a folder or drawer and put them somewhere visible, like next to the person's medications or medical contact information. Be sure everyone in the household is aware of them and knows where they are. You should also make sure the person's doctor has a copy of any documents and is aware of the contents. Surprisingly, this isn't always the case!

It's a good idea to review any directives regularly with the person's doctor. Although a directive that was signed by someone who now has Alzheimer's isn't going to change (that capacity is lost during the moderate stage of the disease), your health team's plan for implementing any stated wishes might shift, especially if there's a new life-changing development like cancer or if the person has become very frail.

Good to know: POLST-type forms can be revised or changed by a health surrogate. A change in circumstances might warrant a different approach.

If there are no advance directives, decision-making generally falls to the person with power of attorney for health care, or absent that, a close relative such as a spouse or adult child. (Rules vary by state.) Past conversations and your personal knowledge about the person can inform those answers to some degree.

You'll want to think beyond medical care to other preferences the person might have expressed or was drawn to that could help him or her to feel loved and at peace now. That can include the people who make appearances during this time, the setting, and what is said and done.

The Conversation Project, a resource dedicated to helping people discuss wishes for end of life care, suggests that in cases of advanced dementia, families can ask, "How would _____ answer this question?" "What mattered most to ____?" (At earlier stages of dementia, the person may be able to participate.) At its website, the Conversation Project provides a downloadable resource for Alzheimer's and other forms of dementia.

Some of its suggested questions, to get you started thinking:

- Would she worry about not getting enough care? Or that she would get overly aggressive care?

- Would she be okay with spending her last days in the hospital? Or would she really want to spend her last days at home?

- Would she want us to take care of all her needs ourselves, or would she want us to get some help from professionals?

- Would she prefer to be alone most of the time? Or would she prefer to be surrounded by loved ones?

- If we had to list the three most important things she wanted us to know about her wishes for end-of-life care, what would they be?

- What was she especially concerned about?

- What was really, really important to her?

- What kinds of treatment would she want (or not want)?

Another key question that's increasingly pertinent: At what point would the person want to back off life-prolonging care?

Admittedly, how hard or easily the answers come depends on many factors. Some of us just "know." Others feel uncertain, especially as circumstances shift. Maybe you've heard your loved one say in the past, "Don't keep me alive once I can't recognize you" (or "if I'm totally bedbound" or "when I don't know where I am" or some other benchmark). Or maybe they always said, "I want you to do everything you can, unless I'm a vegetable." Then it's up to you to translate.

Even written advance directives are still murky terrain when it comes to dementia. Sometimes the language is so vague as to be open to interpretation by families, doctors, and courts. For example, what was a phrase like "extraordinary means" or "unnecessarily prolonging my life" intended to mean?

Some also see an ethical question in whether decisions made while healthy are still relevant if the person appears to want something different when in a cognitively impaired state. One woman, for example, had explicitly told her husband that she didn't want to be kept alive once her Alzheimer's advanced. When she could no longer feed herself, staff at her assisted living facility fed her by hand. The husband felt that she would not have wanted this any more than she would have wanted a feeding tube. When he challenged the action, a court decided she had changed her mind. It ruled that opening her mouth to eat and swallowing indicated a desire to live. Her husband had argued these were mere reflexes, cued by decades of habit.

Consider: What Are the Care Goals?

This is a slightly different question from "What would the person want?" Getting in the habit of thinking in terms of goals throughout dementia care provides you with a useful structure for shaping your decisions, especially toward the end.

"Goals of care" is a catchphrase widely used by health professionals to describe priorities and preferences in a given situation. Thinking through goals of care can help patients and families articulate what's most important for them to get from their healthcare, especially in the context of a serious life-limiting illness.

It's similar to (and indeed fed by) the kind of thinking described in advance care planning, about an individual's values, interests, and vision for the kind of quality of life desired. The difference is that it's an ongoing process. Advance care planning isn't just something that happens (or didn't) when a living will is made. Care wishes then have to be interpreted and applied in actual situations.

This is a new way of thinking for many of us, but an enormously useful and stress-reducing one.

Here's how geriatrician Leslie Kernisan explains "goals of care" to the families she works with: Doctors have three general goals when providing medical care to anyone: 1) to help a person live longer, 2) to help a person function better (for example, walk better or think more clearly), and 3) to help a person feel better (for example, experience less pain, shortness of breath, or fewer uncomfortable symptoms).

Ideally, care satisfies all three, or does so with only minor trade-offs. In some cases, however, these goals begin to conflict with each other. For instance, chemotherapy for cancer might give a person a shot at living longer. It might also cause pain and other side effects, or such fatigue that the person can't walk around as usual.

In Alzheimer's, it's very common for the three key goals to begin to conflict with one another. At some point, being hospitalized may give your loved one a chance at prolonging his or her life, but it will also be likely to cause considerable distress and complications. Or another example: Some families, after conversations with doctors, may decide that the goal of their loved one's medical care will be to avoid hospitalization, because it causes pain and suffering and comes with risks, and instead try to treat infections or other health concerns in the home or nursing home. This plan makes the goal of preserving comfort a higher priority than minimizing the chance of dying.

"Goals of care can be tricky to sort out," says Dr. Kernisan. "You shouldn't try to figure them out on your own. No one is expecting you to."

The truth is you will absolutely need someone with a healthcare background to guide you through one or more conversations about goals of care.

What you can do on your own: Tell the doctors you'd like to discuss goals of care. Even doctors who aren't specialists in palliative care or geriatrics should know what you're talking about or be able to refer you to a clinician who can help you. Another way of getting them to help you explore these trade-offs is to ask about the relative pros and cons of each option you face.

More things to keep in mind:

- Goals change over time as circumstances change.

- Not all goals are strictly medical. They can be personal, focusing on quality of life and how the person would want to live in the time left.

Discussing these goals with the healthcare team means that together, you'll have a better chance at coming up with a medical care plan that's in line with what matters most to your loved one and your family.

Consider: When and How Might You Dial Back on "Usual" Medical Care?

Medical care is good, right? To be sure, we're fortunate to live in a time in which the right medical care can keep us alive longer, make chronic diseases more bearable, and help relieve pain and other uncomfortable symptoms. That said, not all medical care is equally beneficial. Cancer screenings, for example, are designed to benefit people who are likely to live 10 years or more—more than the life expectancy of someone with Alzheimer's. Some forms of medical treatment can even be harmful, especially to those who are frail.

And even beneficial care usually comes with at least some downsides (medication side effects, say, or distress and unnecessary follow-up procedures after a false-positive test result).

Because of all this, specialists often encourage families to consider scaling back on certain forms of medical care as Alzheimer's progresses.

This isn't because they're giving up on the person, or because those with Alzheimer's don't deserve top-quality medical care. Far from it.

Instead, it's because skillful physicians know that the key thing to consider, before recommending a certain form of medical care, is this: *"Do the likely benefits of this medical step* (it could be a drug, a hospital stay, a procedure, etc.) *outweigh the burdens and risks of this intervention?"*

Along with that, they consider a twin question: "Is this intervention in line with person's goals of care, and is it likely to help the person achieve their health goals?"

Geriatricians (doctors who specialize in the health care of the elderly) routinely rely on this helpful benefits-vs.-burdens framework to help families navigate difficult medical decisions or explore options. You can ask those same questions. Health care teams can help you answer them.

No two cases of dementia are exactly alike. One feature they all share, however, is that many common medical interventions will become less and less likely to provide the desired meaningful benefit. So it often makes sense to consider scaling back.

Here are some particular types of medical-decision scenarios that families of someone with dementia are apt to face, according to Dr. Kernisan. Notice how they fall along a continuum:

- *When to pull back from preventative health measures?* Statins, for example, might offer a small reduction in death risk over 10 years, so at some point they're no longer useful to someone with worsening Alzheimer's.

- *Whether to screen for cancer?* Colon cancer screenings, for example, aren't recommended for anyone over age 85, even if there's a history of polyps, because the risk of dying from it is the same whether it's treated or not. If there's dementia, it might make sense to forego screenings at a younger age.

- *Whether (and, if so, how much) to investigate certain symptoms further?* If a simple blood test might confirm a condition that's easily treatable, like an infection for example, and that treatment would improve comfort and functioning, the answer might be yes. If it were an invasive test for a disease with invasive treatment, like biopsying a lung nodule for possible cancer, on the other hand, the answer might be no.

- *When to minimize or avoid hospitalization?* At some point for most people with dementia, a hospital stay is unlikely to improve function or help the person feel better. An aggressive, cure-focused setting no longer makes sense. A study of nursing home residents with advanced dementia described 75 percent of hospitalizations as medically unnecessary or not aligned with the patients' goals (typically, avoiding interventions and being comfortable). Being hospitalized rarely supports a goal of prioritizing comfort for these patients, the authors noted. An exception might include surgery for, say, hip fracture, which can help mobility or the immediate quality of life for some.

- *When to use or forego certain burdensome treatments?* Is using an IV to treat dehydration likely to be successful if the patient wouldn't find it too upsetting? One person might accept it; another might forget why it's there and need to be strapped down, causing upset. What about treatments that are more invasive or intensive?

- *When to use or forego even minimally burdensome treatments?* Treating pain, constipation, and other distressing symptoms is always important. But in the very last stage of dementia, treating something like a urinary tract infection with oral antibiotics may not yield any improvement in function or comfort, or even offer meaningful improvement in lifespan. Many people are receiving hospice care at this point, which can help with these decisions. Medications for dementia symptoms (Aricept, Exelon, Namenda) are another example of treatment that may be moot at this point or even much earlier.

These are all difficult questions. But thinking about them in a context of your loved one's overall health state, balancing the advantages and disadvantages, and knowing that these plusses and minuses evolve according to the situation, gives a framework to help sort through them.

The decisions may not get easier, but you may feel more confident about them.

Consider: How Do You Feel About Where the Death Occurs?

In surveys, most people say they prefer to die at home. In reality only about one in four do from any condition, including Alzheimer's. Most people with dementia still die in nursing homes or hospitals, although more do remain at home than did a generation ago.

Some families choose to bring a loved one home from a hospital or long-term care site at the end of life, with or without the support of hospice, although this can be difficult and isn't common.

Others intend to provide care at home until an emergency (or perceived emergency) upends those plans. One study showed that 20 percent of people with advanced dementia were either hospitalized in the last three days of life or experienced multiple hospitalizations in the last three months. As described in the previous section, these late-life hospitalizations can be incredibly unpleasant for the dying person, not to mention wrenching for families, and expensive.

Still others have strong feelings against a death in their home and hope to avoid it. Or they have culturally guided preferences.

Where the death may occur is a question worth considering early. You may find it harder than you think to find a free bed in a nursing home or stand-alone hospice program, for example. Or, if you intend to keep your loved one home, it's wise to marshal support and know what to expect.

Taking care of someone who's dying is not for the faint of heart. In my experiences, the help of hospice services that were suddenly available at the end of life made caregiving somewhat (emphasis on somewhat) easier. It's still a major responsibility and can be a wrenching experience.

Dementia caregivers have already been treading difficult water for some time, of course. Although we live in an age that's pretty insulated from death, relatives once died at home all the time. Once you go through it you realize there's little that's spooky about it. It's both a sad and extremely meaningful part of life.

Also important to know in advance: who to contact when the death occurs. If the person is enrolled in hospice, it's an easy call, since you'll be given clear instructions. If not, it's a conversation to go over with the primary-care doctor. (See more on this in the section later in this chapter, "At death and right after.")

o o o

SCENARIOS WORTH AVOIDING

Three unpleasant situations can unfold near the end of life almost before you realize that they're happening. They're common yet somewhat avoidable—and therefore worth calling out: the "medical merry-go-round," life support interventions, and a late spike in home-care costs.

The "medical merry-go-round"

It starts when one health setback rolls into another...and another. For example, a bout of pneumonia lands someone with Alzheimer's in the hospital. She's stabilized and discharged to rehabilitation in a long-term care facility. (Medicare covers up to 20 days of the full cost of care in a skilled nursing facility for this, and up to 100 days with partial coverage.) Then she heads home, but within days or weeks another medical crisis lands her back in the hospital.

Each time, the focus is on the immediate "fix." Initial treatment is triggered by good intentions. Families tend to perceive that rehab will improve physical function, experts say. After all, it's the same word we hear when a healthy person breaks a bone or someone has a stroke, leading most of us to agree to or even push for a rehabilitation option. Often, however, this perception contributes to end-of-life care that's rarely curative and can cause tremendous distress. Also common: The normal complications of advanced-stage dementia simply aren't fully explained to the family.

The sad truth is, these "frequent flyer" patients, as the medical community refers to them, tend to get worse, seldom better. More treatment now doesn't equate to better care.

One factor: Hospitalization can lead to "post-hospital syndrome," a general weakness and decline caused by stress, pain, poor sleep, confusion, inactivity, and poor nutrition, or "post intensive-care syndrome" (PICS), a similar problem causing muscle weakness, pain, cognitive decline, and even anxiety or depression.

People with dementia are 20 percent more likely to be readmitted to the hospital within 30 days, compared to those without dementia. Among all adults over 65, CDC data show readmit rates within 30 days already as high as one in five. Among those hospitalized for pneumonia, 12 percent die within 30 days of admission—almost half of these after hospital discharge.

Another hospitalization risk is delirium, an acute change in mental functioning and orientation that more than half of those with Alzheimer's who are hospitalized develop. In most people, delirium's effects are temporary, but studies show that the sharp cognitive declines associated with it can persist for people with dementia. See also, in Chapter 3 under Health Challenges: "Confusion That Suddenly Worsens (Delirium)."

Aside from not getting better, the person spends more of his final days in the confusing chaos of new rooms and new faces rather than in the security and routine of somewhere familiar—often undergoing treatments and procedures they don't understand and that are unpleasant at best and fatal at worst. The whole saga is as stressful on everyone, not least the person with dementia. Ironically, research shows that for the vast majority of those with advanced dementia, families say their primary goal is comfort—which hospitalization, at a certain point, almost always fails to provide.

To help you get through a medical crisis:

For each new situation, pause to think through what the "goals of care" are. Extending life? Adding function? Improving comfort? If all three aren't possible (they won't be, as Alzheimer's worsens), which are most important? Scaling back on life-prolonging care becomes reasonable when the likely burdens on the patient outweigh the likely benefits. That's the point at which helping the person remain as peaceful, pain-free, and comfortable as possible becomes the more desirable and compassionate course of action.

Get medical input on questions that can help you shape those goals. Some conversational starting points:

- Is the condition easily treatable?
- Is the person likely to recover?
- What are the likely side effects of doing this?
- What are the likely side effects of not doing it?
- How stressful will this test or treatment be?
- What would happen if we simply waited and watched this?

Ask the doctor frankly, "How long do you think he or she will live?" Even in late-stage dementia, some doctors are reluctant to be totally candid about what's going on. And it's hard for us, the families, to ask. Mustering the courage and being persistent can help you avoid unnecessary, useless, and uncomfortable treatment.

Ask your doctor for a palliative-care referral. Palliative medicine is a multi-disciplinary approach to medical and nursing care that focuses on comfort over cure. Its goals are to ease suffering from symptoms and improve quality of life, *at any age or stage of illness*. These experts, along with geriatricians, are very helpful at drawing the big picture, helping you understand what to expect, and formulating goals of care.

Someone with dementia is eligible for palliative care at any point after diagnosis. Palliative care teams are present in most hospitals, and some independent private providers exist, but this care can be hard to find outside of big cities.

You aren't likely to get a lot of hands-on help at home. But if your family member is hospitalized or in a health crisis, palliative-care doctors and nurses can help you navigate difficult decisions about pain management, treatments, hospice timing, and other care options. It's their role to consider the whole-person and the big picture, and minimize time spent in the "revolving door" of end-of-life care.

Another newish option to look for: advanced illness management services, sometimes called "pre-hospice." These programs, increasingly offered by health systems, are designed to provide a bridge between curative and comfort care, especially for those receiving care at home.

Beware that there are real problems in the health-care system with "continuity of care"—basically one set of doctors (within a facility or specialty) communicating effectively with another. Palliative care put into place during, say, a hospitalization may not transfer in the records to a skilled nursing facility. So you may have to stay on top of this and ask for repeated consults.

And sometimes the various parties give mixed messages. I'll never forget the distressingly hopeful expression my mother had when her kidney specialist in the hospital triumphantly informed her that a procedure had worked and her infection had cleared. Hooray, except that hours earlier, she'd signed herself into hospice on her oncologist's recommendation because her metastasized cancer had been pronounced untreatable. Such systemic communication problems aside, it's useful to be aware that this level of care exists and that you can ask for it.

Ask if your loved one is eligible for hospice, or when they think it might be appropriate to consider hospice. Hospice is a special form of care for terminal patients; it includes palliative care.

It requires two doctors (typically, the patient's and the hospice's) to certify that the person has less than a 6-month life expectancy if the disease takes its normal course. This can be hard to know with a slow-death disease like Alzheimer's. Still, families don't enlist this care option early enough for people with dementia, and underestimate (or don't know enough about) its many practical, emotional, and spiritual benefits. It's never too soon to at least have a conversation about it.

If your loved one is in a nursing home, hospice will be the first call in a medical emergency, which can circumvent an automatic ambulance ride to the ER, leading to interventions you may not know about or want until it's too late.

Please read the section later in this chapter on Hospice and Dementia.

o o o

Life-support Interventions

Aggressive care for health crises often leads to life-support measures. After all, that's what these external supports—modern medicine in incredible action—are intended to do, sustain life. They were created to maintain vital functions for a short time while the body heals. Someone with advanced Alzheimer's, however, is dying of a terminal illness. Interventions can interfere with this natural process in ways that are uncomfortable and even distressing or painful for the person, potentially prolonging life without enhancing either its quality or the prognosis.

"Doing everything" to live and "dying well" can be at odds with each other.

Interventions in late dementia can include:

- **Artificial feeding** (a feeding tube), used when someone can no longer swallow on their own

- **Artificial hydration** (IV), used when someone can no longer take in liquids

- **Artificial respiration** (a ventilator), used when someone can no longer breathe on their own

- **Cardiopulmonary resuscitation** (CPR), used when the heart or breathing stops

That's not to say these interventions are never appropriate. But for good reason, the pendulum is swinging far back from their use for those with advanced dementia.

Each intervention brings some amount of suffering and risk. Take CPR, for example. It works like a charm on TV hospital dramas, right? In reality, fewer than one in ten people over age 70 survive this kind of resuscitation in the hospital. In 2016, a *JAMA* study that reviewed more than 600,000 cases of patients with advanced dementia who were bedbound found that use of ventilators had nearly doubled between 2000 and 2016, with little change in the death rate (80 percent of the patients died within a year). Artificial feeding can cause diarrhea and infections, and has been shown to offer no advantages over assisted feeding.

What you can do:

Be brave enough to think about these "unthinkable" situations before they happen. Consider what the person would want or has previously articulated a preference for, verbally or in advance directives. Unsure? Ask yourself what you'd want yourself in such a situation.

Or try this: Ask the medical staff what they'd do in your shoes, as a spouse or child, not as an ER doc or a specialist. Many hate that question and are probably trained to sidestep it. But when my mother was dying (of cancer), I pressed her oncologist to be candid with me, her healthcare proxy, about whether he'd choose a particular last-ditch surgery for his own mother, in the same circumstances. His answer echoed what I was feeling in my gut, which was not the option a team of specialists looking only at the narrow issue at hand had offered. I was grateful.

Refusing artificial life support treatments is NOT considered, nor should it be confused with, assisted suicide. It's letting a disease take its inevitable course.

Ask a lot of questions when doctors recommend a treatment: Why is this a good idea? What is the benefit? Will it improve comfort or quality of life, and how? If it will extend life, are there downsides or side effects? How long will this treatment last? Are there alternatives? What will the treatment require of me (the caregiver)? Again, you want to get a good sense of the benefits vs. the burdens in order to make the decision that's in the best interests of the person with dementia.

Ask for help (from a doctor, palliative care consult, or geriatrician) in thinking through the goals of care. It's easy to fixate on the word *life* in "life support" without putting the practices, and their unintended consequences, into a larger context. At a point, giving someone the familiarity of being home with well-managed pain may feel like a more worthy goal than keeping them alive at any cost.

In some cases it may make sense to consider a time-limited trial of a treatment, say a few days, after which you and the doctor can reassess where things stand, Dr. Kernisan suggests.

But know that it's much easier to start an intervention like artificial feeding or mechanical breathing than to withdraw it. (See also: "What About Feeding Tubes?" in the Chapter 3 section on Eating Problems.)

Keep in mind what the normal dying process is like. Fear, denial, and misinformation can be some of the biggest challenges for families struggling with these decisions. Case in point: When someone with end-stage Alzheimer's resists food and drink. Though they're normal, predictable behaviors at this point, they go against our food-is-love, food-is-life human nature. When doing "everything" prolongs dying without enhancing life, however, it's not always the most humane thing.

Many families also fail to realize—until they go through it—that witnessing someone on high-tech life support is more stressful and upsetting than the natural death they often fear.

"What the person with dementia probably needs most is to feel the love and caring of their family. You don't need to keep doing medical interventions to do this," says Dr. Kernisan.

o o o

A Late Spike in Home-Care Costs

Almost a third of Medicare costs are spent during the last six months of patients' lives. The revolving-door syndrome can lead to more co-pays and fees. But even when this isn't the case, someone who's increasingly frail or bed-bound usually has increased personal-care needs at home. If you're physically or practically unable to manage toileting, bathing, and so on yourself, or if you don't want to, you may need to hire reinforcements. It all adds up.

What you can do:

Don't assume you need 24/7 care. When faced with the care of someone bedbound, it might seem essential. If money is no object, go for it. But the cost of all-day, all-night care racks up quickly. In the final stages, the person tends to be in bed or asleep. You're paying a lot for someone to listen to snoring.

If you do hire 24/7 help, it's best to arrange it so you avoid paying overtime for someone working longer than an 8-hour shift or 40-hour week. One silver lining: People who may have been resistant to help or had trouble adjusting to new caregivers earlier in the disease (or fired or flirted with every new face who came along) tend to be much less likely to put up a fuss now, making it easier to bring in multiple new people.

Find someone who will cover just the hours when you need help. Many home-care agencies require you to hire help for a minimum shift of 4 hours or more. But you may only need someone to provide a sponge bath and change sheets, clothes, and incontinence products. Ask if an hourly option with no minimum is available. Or look for an independent caregiver by asking around—your doctor, a care manager, hospice workers, or friends may have suggestions. Some private aides are willing to stop by your home at the end of a shift elsewhere for just the time you need.

Offer to pay more than the going rate, for just the time you need. A four-hour block at $15 an hour will cost you $60. Or you could offer $25 an hour for the help you actually need—to give a bed bath and change sheets, for example.

Lean on friends and family more than ever. This is it. If ever you were going to beg, call in favors, or take others up on their vague offers to help, the time is now.

Shepherding someone through the end of life is a uniquely taxing process. Others who love the person and might like a chance to say goodbye can provide you with needed, no-cost brief respite. Invite them—and don't entertain them when they arrive.

Making specific requests can spur those who are squeamish or unsure how to help. To someone who doesn't want to be in the house: "Can you walk the dog at noon?" To someone who's reluctant to sit bedside: "Please load the dishwasher and take the trash to the curb."

If they refuse, though, accept it and move on to someone else. Some of those who say no are processing their own grief and loss. Some kinds of help may be just too painful for them to shoulder right now. You can burn up a lot of energy judging them and being mad, without changing anything.

Ask about enrolling in hospice care. Most hospice care in the U.S. is paid for by Medicare. Someone with a prognosis of six months or less to live signs a consent form, selecting the Medicare hospice benefit in lieu of regular Medicare benefits. Medicare then pays a set amount to the hospice provider directly, and the hospice program supplies virtually all the people and supplies the patient needs, from care aides and medical staff to medication, incontinence products, equipment, and more.

o o o

HOSPICE CARE AND DEMENTIA

I've separated this out as its own section as a measure of how important and useful I think hospice can be—though it's woefully under-utilized by families caring for someone with Alzheimer's or another form of dementia.

Unlike the word *hospital*, hospice isn't typically a bricks-and-mortar location. It's a philosophy and approach to care, emphasizing comfort and quality of life at the end of life, along with physical, emotional, and spiritual support. It's also a very specific package of benefits. Two-thirds of hospice care takes place in people's homes. The rest is in long-term care settings (nursing homes, assisted living, rehab facilities) or dedicated hospice facilities.

Medicare eligibility requires two physicians (usually the person's primary-care physician and the hospice physician) to certify that the person has a terminal illness with a prognosis of six months or less if the disease runs its normal course. Private insurers also cover hospice but Medicare funds the majority.

I'll be frank: I'm a fan. Both my parents received hospice care (one in their home, the other while in a rehab facility), as did my father-in-law, Don, who lived and died in our home. We requested a hospice evaluation for him after we noticed sudden, upsetting declines in his awareness, mobility, cognition, and disinhibition. He was also sleeping more and declining one or more meals a day—a major change from the man who'd turn up in his dining room chair promptly at 7 am, noon, and 6 pm and never met a cookie or slice of bread he didn't like.

Because of his mostly upbeat emotional state, however, the hospice program was skeptical that he qualified. His HMO suggested bringing him in for an evaluation, but that wasn't practical. It was just too hard to get him anywhere because his strength and balance were so poor. After an in-home evaluation, his dramatic weight loss over the past six months tipped the balance, and he was enrolled in a three-month trial of hospice, which was renewed after his condition continued to decline. He died four months after enrollment.

I know unhappy stories and less-than-ideal hospices are out there. In rural areas, access can be more limited.

Home hospice anywhere still doesn't lift the entire burden of care from families. (Inpatient hospices are easier on families, but availability is more limited.) But on the whole, it's a system that works and brings enormous grace, practical benefits, and stress relief.

As Ira Byock, the pioneering hospice and palliative care physician, once told me, "Trying to care for someone with a serious illness, especially at home, without hospice is like trying to have surgery without anesthesia."

"You can never access hospice too early or stay too late," adds Karen Whitley Bell, a hospice nurse for 20 years in Washington and author of *Living at the End of Life*. "By the final days, there's a limited amount we can do. Earlier is when we can make the biggest difference in managing symptoms and helping people do the things that matter to them." Unfortunately, more than one-third of hospice users miss out because they enroll less than a week before dying. (The median is 18 days.) One in 10 people spends more than six months in hospice.

5 Benefits of Hospice

What's so great about hospice care?

Hospices bring everything needed to the person: a hospital bed, bedside commode, shower chair, wheelchair, medications, bandages, incontinence supplies, expert consults—whatever you need in your specific case. One woman didn't want her husband to die in their bedroom, so the hospice team set up a special room in their house for him. (Hospice care can also be delivered in long-term care facilities.)

Families are privy to a wide range of supports. Home caregivers of people with dementia tend to fall off the healthcare map. There's not much doctors can do, and little home help is available. Hospice suddenly deposits a multi-disciplinary team of aid to your doorstep. A basic team consists of a physician and nurse (both on call 24 hours a day, although you may not see them often), a social worker, a counselor or chaplain, and a volunteer (who will sit with the person, say to talk or read, and provide you some respite care).

Many hospices offer other services as well: personal-care aides, home health aides, music or pet therapists, nutritionists, psychologists, psychiatrists, and occupational, speech, massage, or physical therapists—all of whom come to the home.

You don't have to use all these services. The person may also continue to see his or her regular doctor, though with dementia that's seldom necessary. For caregivers, a huge benefit is that hospice workers and supplies come to you. No more tedious shuttling to doctor's appointments or the pharmacy.

You remain in charge of medical decisions. You decide when to start or stop hospice. If you dislike it, you can quit.

All these backstops tend to lower family stress. The hospice team can show you how to give basic care, talk through the advantages and disadvantages of different types of end-of-life care, provide short-term respite, and offer spiritual or grief counseling to the immediate family—all benefits that go beyond the immediate patient's needs.

Hospice is virtually free. Most hospice is delivered as a Medicare benefit. So you pay only the Medicare premium plus any co-pays or deductibles, which are generally small. Private insurers also cover hospice. Many of your everyday expenses (adult diapers, lotions, medications) disappear.

Hospice manages the aftermath of death for you. One small but critical relief: After the person dies, you only need to make one phone call to hospice. The program then initiates the certifying of the death and removal of the body. Bereavement support is provided for families (including children) while the person is alive and for a full year after the death.

The Challenges of Getting Enrolled

Deciding hospice might be in your family's interests is one thing. Getting it going for someone with dementia can be another story.

To refer a patient to be evaluated for hospice benefits, a physician must certify that he or she has a life-altering condition with an expected prognosis of six months or less. After a referral, hospice evaluates the patient, and then accepts or declines the case.

Determining this may not be easy. Doctors have no biological or scientific crystal ball to predict how long a given patient has left. There's no magic six-month countdown omen (the six-month time frame was picked arbitrarily by Medicare), and doctors are "notoriously bad predictors," says hospice physician Dawn Gross, who hosts the "Dying to Talk" radio program. With dementia, the task is especially tricky.

To determine whether someone is likely to die within six months and certify them for hospice, physicians rely on judgment and Medicare guidelines. For dementia, the leading tool is the Reisberg Functional Assessment Staging Scale (known as the FAST Scale), a 7-stage, 16-level way to describe dementia progression. Stage 6 describes moderately severe dementia—difficulties with basic everyday activities, from dressing to incontinence. Stage 7 is severe dementia. Its sub-stages include being unable to speak more than one word, to walk without help, to sit up unsupported, or to smile.

Medicare hospice eligibility guidelines call for someone to have reached stage 7c (can't walk without assistance) on the FAST Scale and have had one of six other conditions within the past 12 months (pneumonia, septicemia, kidney infection, bedsores, persisting fevers, or weight loss). Complicating the decision for physicians is that these indicators don't accurately predict survival. For example, one study showed that someone who's reached level 7c on the FAST scale (can't walk without assistance) after experiencing all the other FAST stages has a mean survival time of about 4 months, compared to someone at 7c who has skipped earlier steps and might live 10 months.

A person with Alzheimer's can also become eligible for hospice when he or she is in the last stage of another serious condition, like cancer, heart disease, or COPD.

Truth is, families struggling with dementia care could often benefit from hospice-like supports for years. That's currently called palliative care and advanced illness management, two terrific models of care that unfortunately aren't as widely available, or government-funded, as hospice.

That means you'll likely need to be proactive and ask about the possibility of hospice rather than waiting for someone to bring it up first. Let go of concerns that doing so means admitting "defeat" or articulating a death wish. What hospice can add is real comfort for your loved one, with reduced stress for your whole family.

Given how hard it is to prognosticate for dementia, you may also need to be persistent, even insistent, about hospice enrollment if you believe things are taking a turn for the worse. If there seem to be red flags (remember weight loss and functional declines are the two biggies), it's worth asking the primary-care doctor what hospice intake thinks about an initial 90-day trial (the length of the initial benefit). If decline continues, the person may receive a second 90-

day benefit. After that, they're reassessed and re-enrolled every 60 days. In some cases, the person improves—maybe the attentive care helps depression lift and appetite gets better—and they "graduate" from hospice. Indeed, studies show that people often live longer under hospice care than without.

Family caregivers tend to know the individual best. If you're sensing a marked decline, ask about hospice. If you're seeing the signs of end-stage dementia described earlier in this chapter, such as pneumonia or weight loss, ask about hospice.

Don't wait for the signs of active dying (see: "Signs Death Is Very Close" later in this chapter), which typically appear when time is counted in days or hours. To get the maximum help and support from hospice, earlier is best.

Overcoming Common Fears

These are six of the most common concerns I hear about using hospice services at home, along with stress-easing fixes.

1. "I'm not ready to give up."

If you or the doctors are seeing signs of end-stage dementia and the word "hospice" has come up, it only means that the prognosis isn't good, which you probably know in your gut already. The person's body will do what it's going to do.

Contrary to "giving up," providing the attentions of hospice means doing quite a lot, especially in terms of pain management and spiritual and emotional support. It's one of the reasons terminal patients who receive hospice care tend to live longer, on average, than comparable patients who don't.

2. "I don't know what we're in for. Maybe we'll hate it."

Solution: Involve hospice temporarily. Few people know what to expect, because most of us lack a tradition of relatives dying at home. Consider a trial run of hospice. If after a month you're not happy, you can go back to the way things were, even before the initial 90-day benefit ends. You also have a right to change to a different agency once per benefit period.

3. "The house isn't set up right for it."

Hospice can be provided in virtually any setting or circumstance. An initial assessment of the person and the setting will help the hospice program evaluate whatever's needed. They then provide it, so you don't have to shop or figure it out.

4. "I'm worried we might not like the people hospice provides."

You can always ask for replacements, no explanation necessary. Hospices exchange personnel all the time. It can help to let the hospice know whether you're, say, a boisterous, laughing family or quiet types, so they can make a good match.

5. "I don't want my loved one drugged."

It's one of the more persistent myths (based on a few exceptional abuses) that morphine and other medications are used to manage hospice cases literally to death. People who are dying commonly experience pain, anxiety over breathing trouble, and other symptoms. Pain management is part of hospice (and palliative) care, and usually includes opioid painkillers such as morphine, which if needed is started in doses low enough to provide relief without dangerously slowing the breathing rate. Morphine used this way is not a fatal drug.

If it's important to you that the person not be too sedated, let hospice know this preference. Also, know that just because morphine or other meds have been delivered to the home as part of standing orders (routine medications and treatments that can be ordered or begun without contacting the doctor beforehand), it doesn't mean they need to be used.

6. "I'm afraid of the idea of someone dying in my home."

Solution: Get as much info as you can. Ask the hospice you contact if you can talk through these very real and legitimate fears with someone there, as well as with a family who had similar qualms.

Death can be unnerving. Most people find home hospice to be bonding and deeply moving. It's ultimately less about death than about life, your shared life together and a life lived meaningfully until the end.

o o o

SIGNS DEATH IS VERY CLOSE

No one can predict the moment of death, whether from dementia-related causes or any other disease. Certain signs, however, are usually associated with the body's shutting down. As part of the natural dying process, they tell us that the timeframe to the end is more likely days than weeks. These signs can vary in sequence and combination from person to person.

The signs of "active dying" include:

Loss of appetite

Beginning a month or more before death, it's normal to accept only small amounts of bland foods (such as hot cereal), as energy needs decline. Meat, which is hard to digest, may be refused first. Even favorite foods hold little appeal. Then the person will begin to resist or refuse meals and liquids altogether. Someone with very advanced dementia may also be physically unable to swallow.

The medical consensus is that the person isn't suffering or "starving to death." Rather, the body no longer has a need for nourishment or experiences hunger or thirst. The natural dehydration that follows releases endorphins and other brain chemicals that lessen pain and discomfort.

Intravenous (IV) hydration isn't typically given in the active dying stage because liquids may contribute to nausea and the IV can be bothersome to the person. Hydration by hand (such as giving ice cubes to suck or water via water dropper) is standard practice and considered more comfortable. An IV doesn't relieve dry mouth.

Excessive fatigue and sleep

The person may begin to sleep the majority of the day and night as metabolism slows and the decline in food and water contribute to dehydration. He or she becomes difficult to rouse from sleep. The fatigue is so pronounced that awareness of immediate surroundings begins to drift.

Pronounced physical weakness

Activities as basic as lifting the head, shifting in bed, or sipping from a straw become difficult. The person can't sit up without support.

Mental confusion or disorientation

Dying people often seem to be in two worlds at once: here and not here. In the final weeks, they may talk to or gesture toward people who aren't visible to others in the room. Or they may talk about seeing a favorite location, lights, or people living or dead, says British neuropsychiatrist Peter Fenwick, who has studied this. Usually it's people and things connected with peace and security.

"The dying often use symbolic language, especially to indicate an imminent change or a need to go forth—to die," says hospice nurse Maggie Callanan, author of the wonderful book *Final Gifts: Understanding the Special Needs, Awareness, and Communications of the Dying.* Travel is a common theme. The person may allude to "making ready" (packing, making checklists, issuing directions, running late).

Confusion can also be expressed physically, such as by acting restless and picking at bed linens.

Note: The disorientation of active dying can be less obvious in someone with advanced dementia, who may have shown similar symptoms for a long time.

Withdrawal

As the body shuts down, the dying person may lose interest in those nearby. In the final weeks, he or she may speak less often or stop talking, mutter unintelligibly, stop responding to questions, or simply turn away. (Someone with advanced dementia may have long ago stopped doing these things.)

A few days before receding socially for the last time, the dying person sometimes surprises loved ones with an unexpected burst of alert, attentive behavior. This can last from less than an hour to up to a full day.

Labored breathing

In the final hours or days, breath intakes and exhales become raggedy, irregular, and labored. You might hear a distinctive pattern called Cheyne-Stokes respiration: a loud, deep inhalation followed by a pause of not breathing for between five seconds to as long as a full minute—then a loud, deep breath resumes and again slowly peters out.

Note: You might also notice this scary breathing pattern in an older adult who's frail but not dying, due to a condition like sleep apnea or heart failure. A single sign in this list doesn't by itself portend death; most of these signs tend to happen together.

Excess saliva and phlegm in the airway can create loud, gurgling inhalations and exhalations sometimes called "death rattle." Stopped breathing or a wet rattling can be alarming to hear, but the dying person is unaware of this changed breathing.

Changes in urination

Little going in means little coming out. Dropping blood pressure, also part of the dying process (and therefore not treated at this point), also contributes to the kidneys shutting down. The concentrated urine is brownish, reddish, or tea-colored.

Loss of bladder and bowel control may happen late in the dying process. Hospice sometimes decides that a catheter is necessary, although not in the final hours of life. Kidney failure can increase blood toxins and contribute to a peaceful coma before death.

Swelling in the feet and ankles

As the kidneys are less able to process bodily fluids, those fluids can accumulate and get deposited in areas of the body away from the heart. The feet and ankles, especially, and sometimes also the hands, face, or feet, swell or look puffy.

Usually no special treatment (such as diuretics) is given when the swelling seems directly related to the dying process, because the swelling is a result, not a cause, of natural events.

Mottled skin

In the final days to hours before death, skin that had been uniformly pale or ashen develops a distinctive pattern of purplish/reddish/bluish mottling. This is the result of reduced blood circulation. You sometimes see it first on the soles of the feet, but it can show up on the arms, fingers, or other parts of the body. (It looks a lot like bruises.) Nail beds and lips may also look more pale or blue-tinged.

Coolness in the tips of the fingers and toes

In the hours or minutes before death, blood circulation draws back from the periphery of the body to help the vital organs. As this happens, hands, feet, fingers, and toes become notably cooler.

The signs of death listed above describe a natural dying process.

o o o

WHAT ELSE YOU CAN DO

Providing Comfort

It's such a helpless feeling to be a witness to the dying process. Whether or not hospice is in the picture, there are many ways you can ease this transition and express love and support in the final weeks, days, and hours.

What you can do:

If the person is dying at home, ready the bed. Extra pillows can help you establish the most comfort positioning. If you're not already using a waterproof bed pad, it's a good idea to add one. A warm blanket can keep the person comfortable, or he or she may be oblivious. The person may complain about the weight of coverings on the legs, so keep them loose.

Forewarning: Bed linens can become soiled, or you just may not want to keep them afterward. Also, the undertakers who come to transport the body after the death may use the sheets that are on the bed. These are good reasons near the end to try to use bedding—including pillows and blankets—that you don't mind losing. This is not a great time to have heirlooms or fine-quality items in use. It's also wise to be mindful of what the person is wearing, including removing all jewelry.

Focus on physical comfort. Positions that may help breathing: the head slightly elevated with a pillow, sitting up well-supported, or the head or lying body tilted to the side slightly. If there's a lot of phlegm, allow it to drain naturally from the mouth, since suctioning it out can increase its quantity. A vaporizer or a small fan in the room might help. A doctor may recommend oxygen if the person is having breathing distress.

Talk softly or play music. Assume that everything you say can be heard. The sense of hearing is thought to be the last to leave us, even when the person is unconscious, in a coma, or otherwise not responsive.

Favorite music is a wonderful way to fill the otherwise heavy air with relaxation and a kind of emotional sustenance. Don't worry about jazz or 60s rock sounding too upbeat or irreverent for the situation. It's about what brings pleasure now, in this moment like any other.

Permit sleep. The person may sleep most of the day and night.

Avoid jostling the person awake. Speak softly, and identify yourself when you approach.

As appetite ends, don't force-feed. Follow the person's cues even though you may be distressed by a loss of interest in eating. Remember that this, too, is a natural part of dying. Periodically offer ice chips, a popsicle or frozen juice bar, or sips of water for comfort. Try using a water dropper (eye dropper) or syringe to deliver drops of water when swallowing is difficult. Moisten the mouth with a wet cloth or an oral swab stick (a small sponge on a thin plastic handle, sold in drugstores). Moisturize lips with lip balm or petroleum jelly (Vaseline).

Remember the power of nonverbal communication. Even when someone is perfectly healthy, words make up the smallest fraction of the messages we transmit to others. Our tone and body language say most. Hold hands, stroke the arm, snuggle, or hug as you see fit.

Just be there. Given that withdrawing inward is a natural part of the dying process, it's no reflection of your relationship. Maintain a physical presence by touching the dying person and continuing to talk, if it feels appropriate, without demanding anything back. Treasure an alert interlude if and when it occurs, because it's usually fleeting.

Managing Pain

Pain is woefully under-recognized and under-treated at the end of life.

It can have many sources. Someone with dementia may have symptoms from another chronic disease (such as damaged nerves or blood vessels), from dying itself (as breathing becomes difficult, for example), or simply from being bedridden (as muscles atrophy or pressure sores develop). They may also be experiencing emotional pain, including anxiety about what's happening.

Unfortunately, people with dementia often lack the language to express pain. And they may not be able to understand and point to a 1-10 pain scale (even the kind that uses faces instead of words). My dad would wince and clutch his side (he had kidney cancer) but if asked about it, just said on autopilot, "I'm strong like bull!" We learned to watch his body language.

Some indicators of pain in those with Alzheimer's:

- rubbing a limb or other body part

- favoring part of the body

- rapid blinking

- crying

- moaning

- hand-wringing

- using cryptic expressions like, "It's not right." "It's tight." "I don't know what I need."

Seemingly unrelated behaviors like lashing out or restlessness can also indicate pain. My father-in-law grew unusually agitated in his final days. "Jim! I need you! Help me!" he began calling every few minutes for many hours. Responding or holding his hand calmed him only briefly. Two minutes later he'd call out again: "Help me! I need you!" But he couldn't express what he specifically needed. We called the hospice nurse, who stayed for over two hours adjusting his medications to the point where he stopped thrashing and shouting. He was still alert but calm.

Report any signs of distress you see, including changes in behavior, to the doctor. There's a lot that can be done to alleviate unnecessary physical discomfort.

The preferred painkillers at the end of life are opioids, such as morphine or hydromorphone. Let go of concerns triggered by headlines about the nationwide opioid epidemic. Though their potency might seem alarming, when prescribed (or suggested) for a terminal patient, addiction isn't relevant. Morphine is often used in palliative care to manage pain because it acts quickly and is easy to give, orally or in other ways.

These doses won't hasten death, a common fear. What you may notice is that the person may seem "knocked out." This happens because, when released from pain, they're able to relax and sleep. Watch the breathing rate if you're worried. It's not concerning unless there are fewer than 10 breaths per minute. And if you're ever worried, the hospice advice line is there for you 24/7.

You may be asked to dispense oral morphine. If so, a medicine dropper is provided to give a measured dose.

A doctor or nurse will provide a schedule (or tell you what to look for if it's prescribed "as needed," which becomes obvious once you know the signs of discomfort to look for). It's best to drop the slightly bitter liquid directly into the mouth and follow immediately with ice cream or juice to mask the taste. Pain relief comes within 10 to 15 minutes and lasts about 4 hours, longer in someone with diminished kidney function.

Dying people tend to have persistent causes of pain, including arthritis, infection, pressure sores, and breathing difficulty. That's why medication for pain is often given at regularly scheduled intervals throughout the day.

Other drugs may be used according to the specific situation (such as laxatives for constipation, antipsychotics for agitation, or antiemetics for nausea). If you've been wary of antipsychotics earlier in the course of dementia, have an open mind now, because their need and purpose can shift at the end of life.

If you have any concerns, it's definitely fair to ask the same "why" questions about prescriptions at the end of life that should be asked earlier.

Symptom relief can be supported with non-drug measures. An equally important part of palliative care is treating emotional pain, including apprehension and fear, although these can be hard to read in someone with advanced dementia.

Enhancing Life at Its End

Along with basic comfort and medical care, consider things like:

Relationships. Are there particular relatives or friends the dying person would like to see or might benefit by seeing, or by hearing from? For many families, this is an opportunity for closure or reassurances.

Remember that it's very likely your loved one can hear you, even if he or she is asleep, seems "out of it," or may be in a coma. If family members have fallen out of the habit of talking to someone with advanced dementia after they've been unresponsive for a long while, you can reassure them that their connection might matter a great deal now.

Important messages. Hospice workers say it can help to reassure the dying person that you understand and are accepting. In a way, you're granting them permission to set aside the troubles of this world. Even someone with Alzheimer's can benefit from what palliative care physician Ira Byock calls the four core messages, along with "Goodbye," that dying people deeply want, which boil down to: "Please forgive me." "I forgive you." "Thank you." "I love you."

Worried it's too soon for such talk? "It's always too soon, until it's too late," Byock says.

Setting. Being at home means you have greater control over the ambiance, including lighting, temperature, whether windows are open or closed, sounds, how the bed is positioned, and other factors—whether for comfort or cultural reasons. I wish I'd paid more attention to background music in each of my experiences with a dying relative. In hindsight, there was no reason for the solemnity of silence. Music the person loves, whether religious or rock, can be as relaxing or uplifting at the end of life as it is at any other time.

Spirituality. Would the person want to be visited by a clergy member? Have particular final rites administered? Are there prayers, readings, or music he or she might welcome? Although some of us no longer practiced Catholicism, for both of our devout parents, my siblings and I asked a priest to administer the Sacrament of the Anointing of the Sick and Apostolic Blessing ("Last Rites") because we knew it would be meaningful to them.

o o o

At Death and Right After

Is this it? Indicators of death include no movement (including reflexes), no breathing, no pulse, and no heartbeat sound. The pupils don't react to light.

Surprisingly, it's not always immediately clear to a layperson (or even some professionals) when someone has died, especially if breathing patterns have been irregular or the person has been sleeping the majority of the final days. One person might slip away during sleep while another who seemed comatose may bolt upright one last time and open his or her eyes.

In my father-in-law's case, for example, we weren't certain. We'd been on high alert after the hospice nurse who was monitoring him felt that it would likely be a few days at most. Yet he lingered in a here/not here state, mostly asleep, for nearly two weeks. ("I've never seen anything like it," she said.) His breathing, which had been quite shallow for hours, and pulse (or lack thereof) were hard for us to detect.

Finally, after a long period with no movement, my husband and I actually looked at each other quizzically. Because my father-in-law was enrolled in hospice, we called its hotline. The nurse returned to the house within the hour, around midnight, and pronounced him dead. By that point we'd come to the same conclusion.

She then called the mortuary and took care of those details. We also received instructions for all the practical things to do, such as how to dispose of leftover medications and equipment, which was a relief in the strange, numb aftermath when you're left thinking, "Now what?"

Hospice or not, there's no need to call 911 when someone in this situation is dying—or after they die. Emergency personnel are trained to perform CPR and other life-saving measures if someone's heart has stopped. Instead, ask the doctor or palliative care team ahead of time who you should call after death.

If the person is enrolled in hospice, you need only call the number the program provides. If the person isn't in hospice and you don't know who to call, ask the doctor's office. If it's after hours, you can call 911 and inform them that the death was expected, although they may still try to revive the person. Ideally, have Do Not Resuscitate orders you can show them.

Although it's a good idea to have the death certified by medical personnel right away, there's no need to rush. You can spend time with the body or invite a spiritual leader or other family before removal if you prefer.

o o o

SPECIAL STRESSORS NOW

Family Friction

If you've got relatives, you've got differences—of opinion, beliefs, communication style, way of seeing things or doing things—that can run quietly under the surface or flare up in geysers of disagreement. Whatever family dynamics have been around since diagnosis can feel more intense than ever now, for two main reasons:

1) Emotions running higher as death grows imminent.

2) More decision points about care mean more opportunities to disagree.

What helps:

Remember that everyone has a unique relationship with the dying person—and a different way of processing his or her grief. Each family member and friend sees the situation from his or her own point of view. Those who were absent or oblivious throughout the long care journey might be jolted into action now. Some people go into keen denial about death even when it's imminent.

Watching others grieve can be touching or annoying. Reminding yourself that everyone has a different relationship here can stretch your patience, even if it's only a little bit.

Take extra pains to share information with all the relevant parties. With dementia care, the primary caregiver has probably been managing most day-to-day decisions on his or her own. Because of the heightened emotions involved with end-of-life care, it can be especially important now to keep everyone in a more frequent info loop. It helps others mentally prepare for whatever happens, especially if they don't have a front-row seat on providing care now.

Document everything. Save receipts from home-care agencies and Costco runs. Copy and share hospice agreements and medical reports. Taking extra pains to be transparent about finances and other technicalities regarding care can clarify your motives and nip second-guessing by others.

For clashes over difficult decisions, appeal to a third party. One of the most common areas of family discord at the end of life concerns life-sustaining measures like artificial feeding, ventilators, or questionable surgeries. In the absence of advance directives, it can help to appeal to a neutral party you all agree on.

Examples: A palliative care doctor, an aging-life care manager (geriatric care manager), a social worker, a trusted clergyperson, or an elder mediator.

Keep the focus on a course of action. It's polarizing to think that your view is "right" and so the other person's is necessarily "wrong." There are generally few absolute "correct" moves in end-of-life care. In addition to questions like "What's best for Mom?" and "What would Dad want?" it's fair to consider the effects on the primary caregiver. That person's or persons' feelings deserve extra weight.

o o o

Second-guessing Yourself

Everything about end-of-life care is easier said than done. It's straightforward in the abstract and excruciating in the particular. Even if your loved one has signed DNR (do not resuscitate) orders, for example, you may wonder whether this is truly the best course of action in a given situation. A palliative-care team may tell you that a feeding tube won't change the outcome for your spouse and you intellectually agree this is true—but your heart is still pained.

Simply put, it's hard NOT to second-guess yourself as someone's health-care proxy.

What helps:

See the positive side of second-guessing. It means you're conscientiously considering all the angles, including honoring someone's wishes. That ultimately should help reassure you that you've made the wisest decisions you could with the information and advice you had on hand in the moment.

Talk to medical staff or the palliative care or hospice team to get clarity about a decision. The most difficult examples of questioning end-of-life decisions are those to end life-support measures. End-of-life-care professionals can help you see that doing so isn't causing a death; it's no longer artificially prolonging it at a point when death is already inevitable.

Avoid shouldering the full burden of responsibility for decisions. Even if you don't have family members making them with you, you should be guided by medical staff. Another guide, in many cases, is the thoughts and wishes of your loved one that were made and recorded when he or she was of sound mind and body.

See also in Chapter 4: "When You Grieve (Even Though Your Loved One Is Alive)."

o o o

Being There (or Not) at the Moment of Death

It's become something of a tick-box truism for a good death experience, that no one die alone. As a result, there's a lot of unhelpful emotional baggage regarding this. Many people report feeling that they "let down" a loved one by not being there at the exact moment of death. Some even blame themselves as "failures" should this happen, or feel deprived or cheated by having missed this moment. In many cases the survivor had stayed glued to the bedside for hours, determined to be present, turning away or stepping out for only an instant—during which the person passes away.

What helps:

Take counsel from those who work in hospice and have witnessed thousands of deathbed scenes. They believe it's the other way around: Death remarkably often comes minutes after loved ones leave the bedside, as if the dying person were choosing to spare them the final farewell. This is especially true, hospice nurses say, with individuals toward whom the dying person feels protective.

Also common: The dying person seems to hang on to wait for a particular person to visit or something to be said.

Death, like life, turns out to be unpredictable. The measure of your relationship is not reflected or summed up by what happens in its final moments.

o o o

RESOURCES

I can't say it enough: You need all the help you can find. Whether you're just starting down the path of dealing with dementia, or deep into Alzheimer's care, don't miss the following sources of help:

YOUR LOCAL AREA AGENCY ON AGENCY (AAA)

What it is: A government-mandated clearinghouse for general information about community eldercare services. These agencies also offer free referrals to local services that provide transportation, meals, adult day services, in-home caregivers, legal assistance, home-based training programs for caregivers, respite care, and other forms of help.

The names of these agencies often vary by community. But the services they refer to are usually free or low-cost, and calling the agency is free.

How it can help you: Area agencies on aging are one of the best first calls a caregiver can make to learn the local lay of the land on eldercare: what kinds of programs, facilities, and expertise are available to you locally. Staffers can answer common questions and refer you to resources that match your family's specific need—speeding your research process and perhaps making you aware of help you never knew existed.

To find: Start at www.n4A.org. (The "4" refers to the fourth A, as this is the website for the Association of Area Agencies on Aging.)

THE ALZHEIMER'S ASSOCIATION AND SIMILAR ALZHEIMER'S ORGANIZATIONS

What they are: Founded in 1980 as the first national organization devoted to advancing Alzheimer's disease awareness and research, the Alzheimer's Association has local chapters nationwide. The organization also conducts extensive disease research fundraising.

Note: A few local chapters have splintered off from the national Alzheimer's Association, largely over disputes about funding priorities. These just-as-terrific nonprofits offering full-service support include CaringKind (New York City), Alzheimer's Greater Los Angeles, Alzheimer's Orange County (California), Alzheimer's

Texas, Alzheimer's North Carolina, Alzheimer's San Diego, and Alzheimer's New Jersey.

Best bet: Start with the organization closest to you geographically.

How they can help you: Local chapters are a handy way to tap into support groups, educational programs, and other local resources. The national Alzheimer's Association has also partnered with MedicAlert to provide a 24-hour emergency response service for medical emergencies or to find those who wander off.

To find: Start at www.alz.org and also search for "Alzheimer's" and the name of your state or metropolitan area.

ALZHEIMER'S FOUNDATION OF AMERICA (AFA)

What it is: A non-profit uniting more than 2,500 member organizations, including grassroots groups like senior centers, long-term care residences, and home healthcare agencies. Its focus is on education and support both for those affected by dementia and their families.

How it can help you: A main focus is its National Memory Screening Program, a free service offered around the country. AFA's website offers questions to help determine who should be screened and a search for screening sites.

To find: Visit www.alzfdn.org. There's also a toll-free helpline, 866-232-8484.

OTHER LOCAL DEMENTIA SUPPORT GROUPS

What they are: Support groups come in many formats, but most involve small groups of people sharing common experiences under the guidance of a trained expert (such as a social worker or nurse) or a fellow caregiver. They're often held at hospitals, community centers, and places of worship. Participants meet at regular intervals to hear speakers, learn about local resources, and exchange practical ideas and emotional support.

Some groups target spouses, those dealing with a specific stage of dementia, or the newly diagnosed. Groups may be run by hospitals or memory clinics, local Alzheimer's organizations, social-services agencies, or self-starting individuals who are reaching out to fellow caregivers.

A popular new form of support group: "Memory cafes," where people with dementia and their families can socialize. (People with mild cognitive impairment and mild-stage disease find these especially gratifying. Another fast-growing type of participatory program for people with dementia and their families is held at museums, where visitors explore holdings, and sometimes make art too. (In art, there are no "wrong' answers.)

How they can help you: Participating in a support group outside of the home helps caregivers feel less isolated (a common complaint) both physically and emotionally. Others who are going through the same experiences share their stories, mistakes, and successes; strong friendships often form. Groups may feature expert speakers who discuss such relevant concerns as neuroscience, behavioral issues, Medicare, self-care, or family dynamics. Research shows that family members who participate in caregiver support groups report less stress and depression, and they may be better equipped to delay institutionalization of a loved one.

For the participants with dementia, groups are a chance to feel "normal" and involved.

To find: Ask your loved one's doctor for recommendations. Also check community hospitals and local memory clinics or senior centers. For a list of several hundred memory cafes, check memorycafedirectory.com. To find museum-based groups, search "museum dementia programs."

THE ALZHEIMER'S DISEASE EDUCATION AND REFERRAL CENTER (ADEAR)

What it is: Run by the National Institute on Aging, ADEAR is the government's consumer information center about Alzheimer's disease. ADEAR provides research summaries, free publications on memory loss and caregiving in English and Spanish, and general information about Alzheimer's disease.

ADEAR also manages National Institute on Aging-funded Alzheimer's Disease Centers, which are research centers at major medical institutions across the country. In addition, ADEAR manages the Alzheimer's Disease Clinical Trials Database, a joint program of the U.S. Food and Drug Administration and the National Institute on Aging.

How it can help you: The ADEAR's Alzheimer's Disease Centers can be good starting places for creating an action plan to cope with memory loss, especially if you live near one. (They tend to be university-based.) They may offer diagnosis and medical management as well as access to clinical trials of dementia drugs. Participants in clinical trials usually receive free treatment and follow-ups in exchange for helping to advance drug research to slow or cure the disease.

To find: Start at www.nih.gov/alzheimers.

THE BEERS CRITERIA

What it is: Officially known as the Beers Criteria for Potentially Inappropriate Medication Use in Older Adults, this reference lists of more than 50 medications or classes of medications that carry potential risks for people over 65. It was updated in 2015 by a panel of experts in geriatrics. The list was created to help doctors, but anyone can use it.

How it can help you: If the person in your care is prescribed a new medication or you're uncertain about his or her existing drug list, you want to check foremost with the doctor, of course. But if you have any questions, especially if the regular doctor is not a geriatrician, the Beers Criteria is worth a quick check for potential red flags. Listed, for example, are drugs that have a high risk of side effects or limited effectiveness (and better alternatives); medications for common problems that may actually worsen the disorder; and drugs that are best used with caution and careful monitoring.

To find: The American Geriatrics Society offers a PDF of a handy, printable card of these drugs. Go to:

www.americangeriatrics.org/files/documents/beers/PrintableBee rsPocketCard.pdf

THE FAMILY CAREGIVER (FCA)

What it is: The leading non-profit organization supporting long-term family caregivers of all kinds (those caring for anyone from ill children to elders), the Family Caregiver Alliance focuses on education, services, research, and advocacy. Much of what FCA does is "behind the scenes" to the average caregiver: advocating for caregiver-friendly policies, conducting and promoting influential research, working with corporate human-resources officers, and advancing the profile of the growing army of unpaid family caregivers. But the organization also offers many practical services.

How it can help you: FCA's National Center on Caregiving offers tip sheets on such topics as hiring in-home help and a guide to community resources, A resource called Family Care Navigator helps users locate publicly funded caregiver support programs in all 50 states.

To find: www.caregiver.org

MORE ONLINE HELP

The web is ever-changing, and unfortunately, many inspiring dementia blogs don't outlast the caregiver's journey. Here are a few sites and supports worth seeking out:

AlzAuthors

www.alzauthors.com

Don't miss: Archives of the stories behind a remarkable collection of memoirs and more written by spouses, adult children, and others whose lives have been touched by some form of dementia.

Alzheimer's Reading Room

www.alzheimersreadingroom.com/

Don't miss: The robust and always encouraging comments section in the many articles of this #1 Alzheimer's blog site.

Alzheimer's Speaks

www.alzheimersspeaks.com

Don't miss: Radio broadcasts and interviews by advocate Lori La Bey.

Alzheimer's Universe

www.alzu.org

Don't miss: "Everything one needs to know," an interactive teaching tool about disease basics and prevention. While you learn about Alzheimer's, you also help Weill-Cornell Medicine researchers study the impact of public education about Alzheimer's. (Full disclosure: I'm proud to be part of the original Caregiving Expert Panel developing this tool.)

Atlas of Caregiving

www.atlasofcaregiving.com

Don't miss: "Everything one needs to know," an interactive teaching tool about disease basics and prevention. While you learn about Alzheimer's, you also help Weill-Cornell Medicine researchers study the impact of public education about Alzheimer's. (Full disclosure: I'm proud to be part of the original Caregiving Expert Panel developing this tool.)

Don't miss: Downloadable Atlas CareMaps worksheets, which help you identify your support system and resources you may be missing. The Atlas of Caregiving is an innovative effort to find better ways to realistically help family caregivers.

Better Health While Aging

www.betterhealthwhileaging.net

Don't miss: Dr. Leslie Kernisan's detailed articles that teach families how to "think like a geriatrician." You can also subscribe to her Better Health While Aging podcast.

CareLiving

www.careliving.org

Don't miss: The supportive posts aimed at caring for the caregivers by founder Kim Campbell (widow of singer Glen Campbell, who had Alzheimer's).

Daughterhood

www.daughterhood.org

Don't miss: A directory of local "Support Circles" for daughters caring for their aging parents (not just with Alzheimer's), the focus of this group founded by Anne Tumlinson.

Dementia by Day

www.dementia-by-day.com

Don't miss: "16 Things I Would Want If I Got Dementia," a perceptive post by gerontologist Rachael Wonderlin that went viral.

Dementia Mentors

www.dementiamentors.org

Don't miss: Learning about founder Gary LeBlanc's innovative virtual memory café program intended to help those with the disease stay social through confidential 1:1 mentor sessions. Anyone can take part from anywhere.

The Conversation Project

www.theconversationproject.org

Don't miss: The free downloadable starter kit for talking about end-of-life wishes for families of people with dementia.

Make Dementia Your Bitch

www.makedementiayourbitch.com

Don't miss: Nurse practitioner Rita Jablonski's explanation of how fear fuels resistant behaviors. (She's a researcher in this topic area.)

Well Spouse Association

www.wellspouse.org

Don't miss: The extensive local and phone support groups offered by this non-profit for those whose partners have a range of chronic illnesses and disabilities.

The Women's Alzheimer's Movement

www.thewomensalzheimersmovement.org

Don't miss: Brain health advice and stories for caregivers, among the other resources provided by this alliance founded by Maria Shriver to tackle why Alzheimer's disproportionately strikes women.

o o o

HELP ANOTHER HELPER

I'm sorry you've had to join the millions of us who are eyewitnesses to the startling ripple effects of dementia.

I sincerely hope you've found the insights, ideas, encouragements, and practical supports in *Surviving Alzheimer's* to be useful. As I wrote in the book's introduction, I tried to create the resource I wished I'd had at the start of my own experiences.

Wherever you are now in your own caregiving journey, I'd like to suggest three simple "next steps":

1. Go forward from here being kinder to yourself. If there's one takeaway I especially wish readers would hold close, it's that those who care enough to seek out a book like this are tremendously important in this world swamped by the demands of dementia. It's a unique health condition where families and friends, not the medical community, are on the front lines. So thank you for what you're doing.

2. When you no longer need this book, please pass it to a friend or relative. Or donate your print copy to a library, care home, or support group.

3. Kindly post your honest review of *Surviving Alzheimer's* on Amazon or another site. I pay close attention to readers' suggestions to improve future editions. And every positive comment can help convince another prospective reader facing an Alzheimer's experience that there's real help here.

Anything each of us can do to help another is like throwing a life preserver.

o o o

ACKNOWLEDGEMENTS

I love writing lists like this, so I can give credit where it's truly due. At the same time, I hate such lists because I invariably leave off someone I should have included.

I regret, for example, not jotting down the names of everyone who shared a story or an insight with me, over the past six years I've spent writing about aging and Alzheimer's—at conferences and talks, in interviews for articles, in chat groups online and while anonymously exchanging "hugs and prayers" via Caring.com. I've learned so much from my brief encounters with all of them.

Special thanks go to the many aging, caregiving, and dementia experts who inform my work. In the topmost tier, incalculably generous with their time and insights, have been Dr. Leslie Kernisan (especially for her contributions on end-of-life care), Dr. Ken Robbins, and Duke University's Lisa Gwyther.

I'm also grateful to these stand-outs whom I've interviewed or come to know over the years: Dr. Richard Isaacson, Leeza Gibbons, Teepa Snow, Naomi Feil, Bob DeMarco, Amy Goyer, Barbara Kate Repa, Carol D. O'Dell, David Troxel, Joe Matthews, Anne Basting, Joyce Simard, Dr. Gary Small, Mark Warner, Ellen Warner, Geri Hall, Ann Cason, Beth Spencer, Joanne Koenig Coste, Neil Buckholtz, I-Fen Lin, Gail Hunt, Dr. Anton Porsteinsson, Dr. John Morris, Rhonda Montgomery, Dr. Vicki Rackner, Andrea Seewald, Jina Lewallen, Helene Bergman, Suzanne Mogliadini, Linda Fodrini-Johnson, Margit Novack, Gary Joseph LeBlanc, Dr. Dawn Gross, Dr. Eva Selhub, Rafael Romo, Steve Sultanoff, Dave Givens, Jamie Comstock, Guy Eakin, Robert Neimeyer, Maggie Callanan, Dr. Ira Byock, Linda Harootyan, Todd Kluss, Denise Graab, Shoghig Balkian, Bobbi Matchar, Berna Huebner, Mary Mittleman, Darby Morhardt, Dan Cohen, Lori LaBey, and Kim Linder—and I know that's a too-short list.

Among my favorite "real life" experts and sounding boards on caregiving, I count Laura Patyk, Paul Patyk, Mary Gamble, Patti Anderson, Beth Hanes, Kay Strom, Brenda Avadian, Susan Morris, Frank Winckowski, Amy Keller, Rhonda Swink, Jamie Blackmon, Santa Bogdon, Jamie Gannon, Bob Rachlow, and Barbara Haynes.

Helpful groups that contributed to this project include the Gerontological Society of America and New America Media, which together administer the Met Life Foundation Journalists in Aging fellowships; the National Press Foundation and its Alzheimer's Disease Issues journalist training program; the Journalists Network on Generations (and its tireless creator Paul Kleyman), the Family Caregiver Alliance, the Alzheimer's Foundation of America, and the Alzheimer's Association.

I also want to thank those who helped me with production and design: Allyson Appen, Jonathan Tuttle, and Margaret Spencer.

Not last or least to be acknowledged—more like first and foremost— is Jim Scott, my partner in business, in caregiving, and in life.

Thank you, all.

o o o

ABOUT THE AUTHOR

Paula Spencer Scott writes, speaks, and consults about women's life-stage challenges. Active in caregiver education, she created the popular "Steps & Stages" Alzheimer's resource for Caring.com (where she was a contributing editor and launched its Alzheimer's channel) as well as curriculum for Weill-Cornell's Alzheimer's Universe (AlzU). She's currently developing an online course for families caring for someone with dementia (see survivingalz.com).

An award-winning columnist for *Woman's Day* and *Parenting* magazines and a fellow of the Gerontological Society of America's Journalists in Aging program, her work also appears in *Parade*, *AARP Bulletin*, *Next Avenue*, *WebMD*, and elsewhere. Her 13 books include *Like Mother, Like Daughter*; *Momfidence*; and the collaborations *The V Book*, *Bright From the Start*, and *The Happiest Toddler on the Block*. Five close family members have had dementia.

Paula's website for dementia caregivers: survivingalz.com

Follow her on Twitter: @PSpencerScott

Like Paula's *Surviving Alzheimer's* page on Facebook here: facebook.com/survivingalz

Send your feedback to survivingalz@gmail.com

o o o